Shoulder impingement syndrome: The role of imaging modalities

Dr. Sabah Hasan Shindakh Nooralden, MBChB
Director General Directorate of administration, regulation and finance
Iraqi Ministry of Health
Baghdad, Iraq

ISBN-13: 978-1729543641
ISBN-10: 1729543642

Copyright 2018 © Iraq Headquarter of Copernicus Scientists International Panel

Content	
CONTENT	3
PREFACE	4-5
CHAPTER ONE	
SHOULDER IMPINGEMENT SYNDROME	6-17
CHAPTER TWO	
CLINICAL DIAGNOSIS OF IMPINGEMENT SYNDROME	18-25
CHAPTER THREE	
SHOULDER ANATOMY	26-33
CHAPTER FOUR	
IMAGING DIAGNOSTIC MODALITES: PLAIN FILMS (X-RAYS, RADIOGRAPHS)	34-44
CHAPTER FIVE	
IMAGING DIAGNOSTIC MODALITES: ULTRASONOGRAPHY	45-73
CHAPTER SIX	
IMAGING DIAGNOSTIC MODALITES: COMPUTED TOMOGRAPHY	74-75
CHAPTER SEVEN	
IMAGING DIAGNOSTIC MODALITES: MAGNETIC RESONANCE IMAGING	76-112
CHAPTER EIGHT	
TREATMENT OF SHOULDER IMPINGEMENT	113-116
CHAPTER NINE	
THE ROLE OF SHOULDER IMAGING IN DIAGNOSIS, STAGING AND MANAGEMENT OF SHOULDER IMPINGEMENT	117-121
ACKNOWLEDGEMET	122
BIBLIOGRAPHY	123-150

Preface

This book represents a thesis entitled "Shoulder impingement syndrome: The role of imaging modalities in diagnosis, staging and management" .The thesis was submitted by Dr Sabah Hasan Shindakh to the College of Medicine, University of Granada in the partial fulfillment of the requirements for the degree of Master in diagnostic and therapeutic radiology and physical medicine.

The thesis was supervised by Dr. Fernando R. Santiago. The evaluation committee of the thesis included Professor Doctor Jose Luis Martin Rodreiguez, Dr Serran Olea Necolas, and assistat professor, doctor Mariana Fatima Fernandez Cabrera.

The aim of the thesis was to evaluate and compare the relative advantages of each imaging modality in their ability to aid in the diagnosis, staging and management of shoulder impingement syndrome.

The thesis studied the role of imaging modalities in diagnosis, staging and management of shoulder impingement syndrome, and concluded that imaging is a core component of the diagnostic process which also includes appropriate history and clinical examination.

Plain radiography was considered the first line of imaging, and can provide very useful information on the shoulder anatomy. However, the inability to visualize occult signs and soft tissues such as tendons and muscles limits its usefulness in diagnosis and staging.

Ultrasonography is the second line of imaging, and is effective in diagnosing several rotator cuff pathologies and non-rotator cuff diseases.

Ultrasound can accurately stage rotator cuff disorder and assess the volume of muscles of the rotator cuff. Dynamic Ultrasonography has diagnostic qualities not present in other imaging modalities, making it very useful in the diagnostic and staging process.

Computed tomography provides an excellent visualization of joints post-trauma, and can help in prosthesis management or surgical planning.

Computed tomography scans are also very useful in evaluating glenoid rim fractures and shoulder dislocations.

Magnetic resonance imaging is considered the gold standard for imaging shoulder dysfunction. Although expensive, it has many advantages including reliability, comprehensiveness, non-invasiveness, lack of radiation and ability to visualize soft tissue.

MRI scans can make images in all three dimensions and provide detailed pathology that is invisible other imaging modality, such as inflammation and fluid accumulation.

MRI imaging also has an important role to play in treatment, as it can assess tissue damage and determine how well a patient will react to surgical intervention (or whether a non-operative approach might be better suited).

When deciding which modality to use, doctors must balance the benefits, the risks, the cost, the appropriateness and the available resources. This book provides an in-depth examination of these factors, and provides a template for clinicians to use in their daily practice.

CHAPTER ONE: SHOULDER IMPINGEMENT SYNDROME

Shoulder impingement syndrome is a condition which includes a variety of symptoms, typically caused by inflammation and/or degeneration of the supraspinatus tendon as it passes through a narrowed subacromial arc. The condition is not a pathologically-consistent diagnosis, and represents a spectrum of shoulder pathologies with various mechanisms and etiologies.

The term "subacromial impingement syndrome" is commonly used to describe a group of conditions including subacromial bursitis, partial tears and rotator cuff tendinopathy.

Shoulder disorders are commonly classified according to three metrics:

1-The anatomy of the disease (rotator cuff disorder or subacromial pain syndrome). Rotator cuff disease or disorder is a multi-factorial syndrome resulting from a number of internal or external factors.
2-The underlying mechanism (tendinosis, rupture or tendinitis).
3-The etiology (repetitive sprain or work-related).

Impingement syndrome is not a specific diagnosis as it includes several disorders having similar presentations, and associated with a comparable constellation of symptoms, and covers several rotator cuff pathologies. The current definition of impingement is a description of a presentation, and dose not represent one diagnosis.

However, the recent improvements in diagnostic tools allowed the replacement of this non-specific term with a number of more accurate diagnoses which provides a better description of the individual causes and mechanisms of impingement syndrome.

The variability in the term 'impingement syndrome' also varied by specialty.

Radiologists generally describe impingement syndrome according to the morphology and anatomy,

Orthopedists consultants generally describe the condition simply as impingement.

Industrial medicine practitioners generally describe the condition in terms of etiology (such as being work-related).

Variation in diagnostic criteria has created difficulties in treatment and research.

Treatment can become inappropriately branched without diagnostic consistency. When the diagnosis is motion-based, physical therapy will be the predominant treatment; when the diagnosis is anatomically-defined, treatment will likely be surgical.

Experts have suggested that the term "Impingement syndrome" should be broken down. The symptoms of the disorder should referred to as "antero-lateral shoulder pain", whilst the anatomical aspects of the disease should be classified as "rotator cuff disease or disorder".

INCIDENCE AND PREVALENCE

Shoulder impingement can be a potentially debilitating condition and associated with a significant impact on a patient's quality of life.

The disorder generally has a gradual onset, often progressing to a chronic or recurrent presentation. The condition frequently affects working-age patients, and therefore it has a significant economic impact in industrial countries, both through loss in productivity and the costs of its treatment.

Shoulder pain has been considered as one of the most common musculoskeletal symptom that patients present with. It either comes second or third in the rankings (depending on study), along with lower back pain, knee pain or neck pain.

In some studied, shoulder pain accounted for around 1-3% of all visits to doctors. Some studies found that around 7% of the population present with shoulder pain annually. However, this figure can rise to up to 14% in working-age populations.

Shoulder impingement syndrome is the most common cause of shoulder pain in a primary healthcare setting, and was accounted for 44-65% of all shoulder pain presentations in some series.

The prevalence of shoulder pain was estimated to be between 7% and 31%, and is much commoner in the elderly population.

The prevalence of new-onset shoulder pain peaks in women aged 50-59 and men ages 60-69. It was estimated that around 50% of the general population can experience a single episode of shoulder pain in the course of a year, and around 10% will present to the doctor over the course of their lifetime. Around 1-2% of individuals over 18 present with shoulder pain annually.

However, it is estimated that only 20-50% of patients experiencing shoulder pain will ever consult a clinician. In the United Kingdom, around 2.4% of all GP visits were for shoulder pain, whilst in the United States they accounted for around 4.5 million presentations.

Over 300,000 rotator cuff surgeries were performed in the United States every year, and the management of patients with shoulder pain costs up to 3 billion USD.

CAUSES AND PATHOLOGY

Shoulder pain may arise from muscles, bones, tendons, bursae and nerves.

The etiology of shoulder impingement syndrome has been attributed to two competing theories: intrinsic (degenerative) and extrinsic (mechanical).

This dichotomy can also be parsed as structural/functional or intra-tendinous/extra-tendinous.

Neer (1972) suggested that the most prevalent cause of impingement syndrome is the extrinsic impingement of the acromion.

However, recent improvements in the quality of imaging especially arthroscopy provided patho-anatomical evidence are in favor of the intrinsic theory.

The cause of shoulder impingement is more likely to be complex and multi-factorial and include external compression, degeneration of old-age and vascular insufficiency.

The term "Primary impingement" has been used to describe a shoulder disorder that occurring in isolation. The term "Secondary impingement" has been used to describe the condition accompanied by other problems such as AC issues, instability or calcifying tendinitis.

The extrinsic causes of impingement can be divided into two main categories:

A-Anatomical factors including acromion shape and AC degeneration.
B-Biomechanical factors including scapular kinetics, humeral kinetics, postural issues, muscle deficits, and soft tissue tightness.

ANATOMICAL FACTORS

Any pathological process that causes a disturbance in the subacromial structures can cause impingement of the shoulder.

There are a number of morphological variations of the acromion and pathologies of the AC joint (osteophytes, bone spurs) that can cause compression of the subacromial area, which in turn causes impingement.

Narrowing of the subacromial space can result from:

Longstanding inflammation of the subacromial bursa.
Calcification of the coraco-acromial ligament.
Fracture of the proximal humerus.

Shape of the acromion

Neer's theory of extrinsic causation of impingement has been widely accepted. Neer theory suggested that inflammation and irritation of the subacromial tissues is the underlying cause of pain in impingement.

In rotator cuff disease or disorder, tendons are mechanically impinged below the inferior layer of the anterior third of the acromion and the AC joint.

Difference in the structure of the coraco-acromial arch can cause discomfort, and this difference can result rotator cuff injury.

A study examined the architecture of the coraco-acromial arch in impingement patients; found that a normal architecture was present in 6%, whilst 46% had an aggressive arch. Another study reported that 50% of rotator cuff tendinitis patients had Type 1 acromions, whilst 58% of full-thickness rotator cuff tear patients had Type 3 acromions.

A wide variety of structural associations with shoulder impingement syndrome have been observed including:

The shape of the acromion.
Variations in the acromio-clavicular joint.
The attachment of the coraco-acromial ligament.

Bigliani and Levine (1997) has categorized this acromion changes according to their propensity to cause impingement syndrome, with Type 1 associated with the lowest incidence of impingement and Type 3 associated with the highest incidence.

A Type 1 acromion is generally flatter in shape, Type 2 is more curved (lying parallel to the humeral head), and Type 3 has the appearance of being hooked which may then impinge on the rotator cuff when the arm is raised.

It has been suggested that individuals with a Type 3 acromion are at an increased risk of developing shoulder impingement.

The correlation between acromion shape and rotator cuff rupture could be explained independently by increased incidence of both factors with increasing age; the older the patient, the more likely they are to have both Type 3 acromion and rotator cuff ruptures.

It has also been suggested that the severity of impingement syndrome is associated with the architecture of the acromial arch.

Degeneration of acromio-clavicular (AC) joint

The acromio-clavicular joint contains an intra-articular disc susceptible to degeneration with age or because of trauma resulting in degeneration of the surrounding joint, leading to degenerative arthrosis.

Neer suggested that progressive deterioration of the AC joint can cause impingement. The rotator cuff tendons come into contact with the AC joint when the gleno-humeral joint is abducted 60°. When the joint is abducted by 70° the greater tuberosity is directly below the AC joint; when the joint is in this arrangement it only requires a small narrowing in order to cause inflammation of the rotator cuff.

Rotator cuff tears are also correlated with inferiorly directed osteophytes in the presence of AC space narrowing and subacromial impingement.

Pain resulting from this sort of AC pathology tends to be particularly resistant to the standard impingement therapies (acromioplasty, coplaning).

Coraco-acromial ligament

The coraco-acromial ligament can also cause impingement syndrome. When the gleno-humeral joint is forwardly elevated or internally rotated the coraco-acromial arch comes into contact with the rotator cuff.

Neer (1972) suggested the existence of an association between coraco-acromial arch anatomy and impingement syndrome. It has been reported that both coraco-acromial ligaments with several bundles with long lateral borders and large coracoid insertions are associated with rotator cuff tendon deterioration. There is no indication that rotator cuff degeneration is associated with the type of coraco-acromial ligament.

Osacromiale

An osacromiale occurs when the epiphysis of the anterior end of the acromion fails to fuse. An osacromiale joint may become unstable or tilt anteriorly because it is attached to the coraco-acromial ligament, and cause impingement.

Osacromiale is fairly rare as a lone condition. When seen in imaging, it tends to be an incidental finding. Studies have suggested varying figures, but the incidence is estimated to be between 1.3% and 1.5%. Impingement that results from an unstable osacromiale is very uncommon, and it is much more likely that osacromiale will be present in a coexistent rotator cuff tear.

Subacromial bursa

Impingement can also occur when the subacromial bursa becomes inflamed, and reducing the volume of the subacromial space. This diagnosis can be tested for by injection a local anesthetic into the local area.

Coracoid impingement

Coracoid or sub-coracoid impingement is much less common than subacromial impingement, and therefore it is often missed. In coracoid impingement, the tendon of biceps or subscapularis is compressed between the humeral lesser tuberosity and the coracoid process.

An association between the presence of anterior shoulder pathologies and sub-coracoid stenosis or a narrowed coraco-humeral distance has been suggested. However, there is no consensus on the validity of coracoid impingement as a diagnosis, and what its therapeutic criteria.

Intrinsic causes of impingement syndrome which cause changes to the tendons of the joint can be a result of variance in the followings:

Biology (degeneration, the aging process, a reduced blood supply).
Mechanics (overuse, tensile or shear overload, trauma to the area).

Most recent evidence is in favor of the intrinsic theory of rotator cuff disorder.

The intrinsic causes of disorder include:

Age-related degeneration.
Insufficient blood supply.
Tensile overload.

Changes in the matrix of the tendon.
Genetics: The role of genetics as an integral factor in the health of the shoulder joint has been suggested.
Muscle dysfunction: Intrinsic tension overload of the affected has been suggested as the predominant cause of rotator cuff tendinitis.
Overuse of the shoulder resulting in inflammation and thickening of the bursae or tendons can cause impingement.

Rotator cuff tendinitis may occur in acute or chronic inflammation caused by overuse (intensive work, heavy lifting, and awkward posture), irritation, strain, poor mechanics or micro-trauma; regardless of cause, the disease tends to be progressive in nature.

The inflammation caused by these changes results in a reduced subacromial space. This narrowing of the subacromial space results in edema and tendinitis in the area with soft tissues occupying an increasing volume of the subacromial space and causing increasing friction against the coraco-acromial arch.

Overuse of the joint is commonly reported in athletes who perform a sport involving an overhead arm motion.

Aging may be associated with poor regeneration associated with local inflammation, and pain around the tendons of the shoulder.

Degenerative tendinopathy

Ogata and Uhthoff (1990) suggested that the predominant pathology of partial rotator cuff tears is tendon degeneration. They also suggested that degeneration can cause proximal migration of the head of humerus, resulting in both impingement and complete cuff tears.

Internal impingement

Of the biomechanical factors, internal impingement is distinct from the traditional extrinsic causes of the condition. It is instead caused by compression of tendons between the glenoid and the head of humerus.

Internal impingement is a complex condition, and occurs most commonly in athletes who practice sports involving a throwing or overhead movement of the arms.

The condition is associated with certain specific phases of motion: repeated abduction and external rotation of the arm. This movement causes recurrent contact of the postero-superior-glenoid with the humeral greater tuberosity. However, it was thought that this contact of glenoid and humerus could be physiological rather than pathological.

Repeated contact may cause fraying of the articular rotator cuff tendons and lesions in the postero-superior-labral region.

STAGES OF IMPINGEMENT

Neer (1983) used a staging system for impingement, covering the disease from tendinitis and fibrosis to a partial or complete rotator cuff tear.

Neer stated that this disease process is a spectrum, with rotator cuff tears being an end-result of longstanding impingement. Shoulder impingement may be a reversible inflammation of the area, or it may be full rupture of the cuff accompanied by significant degeneration.

Stage I impingement presents with edema and bleeding, typically observed in patients under twenty-five years.

Stage II impingement is characterized by fibrosis and tendinitis of the cuff caused by recurrent inflammation. This stage is typically noted in patients aged 25-40 years.

Stage III impingement is the chronic stage of the disease, with partial or full tears of the cuff, and is generally only observed in individuals older than forty years.

RISK FACTORS

Risk factors for impingement syndrome that increase the incidence regardless of etiology include:

Aging

The older the patient, the greater the incidence of shoulder pain. However, age tends to have a larger impact on rotator cuff disorder than on shoulder pain.

Age is also significantly correlated with AC joint degeneration and medial acromion sclerosis.

As with other shoulder pathologies, the incidence of both symptomatic and asymptomatic rotator cuff tears (partial and complete) increases with age.

It is common for individuals with asymptomatic cuff tears to develop pain or discomfort over time. In patients younger than 18 years, the predominant cause of shoulder pathology is gleno-humeral instability. It also appears that the presence of a Type 3 acromion, in the absence of other causative factors, does not result in shoulder impingement.

The number of presentations also rises over the course of a patient's working life, but fall following retirement. However, older patients have significantly poorer recovery rates than younger ones.

Sex

Female tend to have a higher incidence of musculoskeletal issues than men especially for neck and shoulder problems. This trend is also present in shoulder pain. This difference in incidence was not attributed to age, level of education, weight, fitness, or smoking status.

Hand dominance

Shoulder impingement syndrome is strongly associated with the dominant arm of the patient. Chronic shoulder syndrome occurs in the right shoulder in about 5% of the population, and in the left shoulder in 3%.

The Health 2000 Survey reported a twofold discrepancy between right and left arms in working age populations, strongly implying a correlation between the syndrome and physical movement. It has also been suggested that the presence of shoulder impingement in one arm increases the risk for developing it in the other arm.

Work

There are a number of work-associated causes for impingement including:

Repetitive manual labor.
Overload of the joint.
Forceful movement.
Prolonged static loading.
Working with arms elevated above the level of the shoulder especially with tools.
The presence of vibration on the arm.
Repeated arm abductions.
Ergonomics of a particular job: It has also been reported that the more years of education a patient has had, the less likelihood of a patient developing rotator cuff tendinitis or have chronic shoulder pain. The Health 2000 Survey found that this trend applied to both men and women.

The incidence of shoulder problems is increased with the following factors:

Intense physical or psychological demands.
Lack of job control.
Low skill level.
Poor supervision and prior work stress.
Perceiving the job as being stressful and feeling unsupported was associated with significantly poorer shoulder recovery.

Psychological and psychosocial factors

The incidence of shoulder pain is higher in patients experiencing excessive mental stress and has poor social support.

Poorer psychological health has also been correlated with a longer course and poorer prognosis of shoulder disorders.

A British cohort study (Macfarlane, et al, 2009) reported increased prevalence of shoulder pain in the lower the socioeconomic status which was attributed to lifestyle factors, adverse life vents, increased stress and poor mental health.

A Dutch cohort study (Reilingh et al, 2008), and Bot et al, 2005) showed correlation between mental health and shoulder pain.

This link between mental health and shoulder pain works in both directions. Patients who suffer from generalized or non-specific pain are likely to suffer from alexithymia, depression and burnout.

These effects have a knock-on impact on almost all aspects of a patient's life: those with impingement have poorer health outcomes and a lower quality of life than the general population.

Pain catastrophising can determine how pain is perceived and how a patient manages it. This, in combination with community, experiential, cultural and genetic factors, can drastically worsen pain.

All of these aspects must be considered when creating a care plan for a patient with impingement.

Without proper explanation, patients may resort to completely immobilizing the arm, and worsening the pain in the long term. Patients should be encouraged to move and perform usual activities, even if pain is present.

Obesity with a larger weight circumference is associated with a higher risk of developing shoulder problems, most notably rotator cuff tendinitis. However, some studies have failed to demonstrate a link between obesity and shoulder pain.

Diseases including strokes, Parkinson's and diabetes, have been reported to increase the risk of shoulder problems.

CHAPTER TWO: CLINICAL DIAGNOSIS OF IMPINGEMENT SYNDROME

The classical presentation of shoulder impingement includes a dull ache worsening progressively over several weeks.

The pain generally localizes to the antero-lateral region, radiating to the lateral humerus. The pain is generally worse at night, often waking patients up if they lie on the affected arm, or if they rest the arm above the shoulder. About 89% of patients report night pain.

Pain is worse on resisted abduction. These symptoms interrupt daily activities, especially one which require certain movements of the affected shoulder such hair combing, reaching round one's back, raising one's arms.

The painful arch presents clinically with painful abduction, and is associated with a reduced range of movement, arm power and functional capability. Although weakness and stiffness are often present, these symptoms are usually a result of the pain. Shoulder impingement can often become chronic, with recurrent, intractable pain. About 40% of patients continue to experience pain a year after diagnosis.

The clinical examination is performed after taking a full clinical history including:

Features of the pain (site, onset, character, radiation, associated factors, duration, exacerbating or alleviating factors and severity).

Associated symptoms such as stiffness, weakness and instability.

Physical examination includes inspection, palpation and movement of both shoulder joints.

The relevant abnormalities on inspection and palpation include scars, wasting, deformities, asymmetry, posture, erythema and warmth.

Movement can be tested both passively and actively. The following movements should be assessed: forward elevation (flexion), extension, abduction, crossbody adduction, external rotation and internal rotation.

Assessing shoulder abnormality demands a comprehensive approach a myriad of causes have to be considered.

DIAGNOSTIC CLINICAL TESTS INCLUDE:

Neer's test to detect **Neer's impingement sign** which is detected when the arm of the patient is passively elevated with the patient seated and the examiner standing behind him or her.

As the acromion and clavicle are pressed down upon, scapular rotation is reduced. Flexion of the arm pushes the humeral greater tuberosity below the acromion. As this occurs, the supraspinatus tendon becomes compressed between these two structures; in an impingement patient, pain will be elicited.

The pain occurs because the supraspinatus tendon comes into contact with the acromion and coraco-acromial ligament, and the greater tuberosity of the humerus. Internal rotation increases the contact force, and pain.

This test can be confirmed through the application of local anesthetic to the area below the anterior acromion: if this relieves the pain, it is impingement. The sensitivity of this test is between 75% and 89%.

The painful arch test is performed with the patient standing and actively elevates and lowers the arm in the abducted position. If there is pain at 60° and 120°, the test is considered positive for impingement.

Hawkins-Kennedy test is performed with the patient standing opposite the clinician and flexing their arm to 90°. The clinician passively internally rotates the arm and lowers it. This motion puts the interior aspect of the coraco-acromial ligament in contact with the humeral greater tuberosity and causes impingement upon the supraspinatus tendon. The test is positive if the scapula rotates or the patient reports pain.

The Hawkins-Kennedy test is 92% sensitive, and is associated with a different mode of impingement to the Neer's test.

Yocum's test is performed with the patient to resting the hand on the opposite shoulder; the clinician then lifts the elbow but keeps the shoulder in place. This produces a similar physiological response to Hawkins test, and is positive if there is pain.

Cross-body adduction requires the arm to be forwardly flexed by 90°, and then adducted across the torso; this causes AC compression, and pain in impingement.

Jobe's test which is also called the "empty can test" is performed with the patient actively elevates the arm with the elbow in full extension. The patient then fully internally rotates their arm with their thumbs down (in the plane of the scapula. This test assesses the supraspinatus tendon. If there is pain or weakness when the movement is resisted, the test is positive.

Codman's sign which is also called the "drop arm test". The patient starts the test with their arm in full abduction; they must then gradually adduct their arm in the same manner. If the arm suddenly drops, the test is positive. The test assesses weakness or pain in the supraspinatus tendon, and has a specificity of 97%.

The infraspinatus drop sign is performed with the clinician to maintaining the patient's arm at 90° elevation (in the scapular plane). The arm is externally rotated and the elbow is flexed to 90°. If the patient cannot maintain this position and uses the infraspinatus muscle, the test is positive.

The strength of the infraspinatus muscle can be tested by positioning the patient with the arms along their torso, and the elbows flexed at 90°. The patient's arms are then passively internally rotated against resistance; this allows the clinician to evaluate the relative strength of each infraspinatus.

The external rotation lag sign measures the integrity of infraspinatus and supraspinatus. The examiner stands behind a seated patient, with the patient's arms at 90° flexion. The examiner raises the arm by 20° in the scapular plane whilst externally rotating the arm. The examiner then releases the wrist whilst holding the elbow. If the patient cannot keep the arm externally rotated (and the arm drops), the test is considered positive.

Gerber's test which is also called the lift-off test. The patient puts the hand on the back at the level of the waist, with the arm internally rotated and the elbow flexed at 90°. The examiner pulls the arm 5-10cm off the back, and keeping the arm in the aforementioned position. The patient attempt to maintain this position without support. In the presence of weakness, the arm jumps forward against the back. This positive sign signifies rupture of the subscapularis tendon.

The Gilcreest palm-up test is performed with the patient actively raises the arm with the palm face-up and the elbow in extension. If pain is present in the anterior arm when there is resistance, the test is positive. This is not a test of power, but instead elicits pain in the long head of the biceps.

A review of the relevant literature suggested that several of these tests (Neer's, Hawkins and Neer injection) were very sensitive, but not specific.

The external rotation resistance sign and painful arc test are considerably more specific for rotator cuff disease.

The Cochrane Database of Systematic Reviews suggested that there is a great diversity in the type and value of shoulder impingement tests. The Cochrane Database also suggested that any one test was not sufficiently accurate for it to be suitable in diagnosis of impingement. Therefore, it is recommended that physicians use a combination of tests in order to confirm the diagnosis. For subacromial impingement, the following tests are most suitable: Hawkins, the painful arc test and the infraspinatus muscle strength test.

CLINICAL PRESENTATIONS OF INTERNAL IMPINGEMENT

Internal impingement is a syndrome associated with repeated and excessive friction between the posterior-superior-glenoid and the posterior humeral head, present when the arm is abducted and externally rotated in extreme.

It is very difficult to diagnose internal impingement based on a history in isolation, as the presenting symptoms are relatively nonspecific, shared with several other shoulder conditions.

The following symptoms tend to be present in a large proportion of internal impingement patients:

Diffuse pain in the posterior shoulder girdle, but occasionally localized to the joint line. This presentation is particularly common amongst athletes of throwing sports. The pain is worse during the late-cocking phase of throwing (arm at 90° of abduction in external rotation).

Acute pain following inciting incident tends to present in athletes from non-throwing sports.

Decrease in throwing velocity with gradual worsening in the throwing speed and deteriorating control of the movement; most noticeable in overhead-throwing athletes.

Dead arm with the sensation of arm and shoulder weakness following throwing, accompanied by a subjective feeling of shoulder slipping.

Asymmetry of the muscles between the non-dominant and dominant shoulders presents in overhead throwers.

Muscular/Neuromuscular imbalance in the muscles of the shoulder and poor control of the scapula.

Increased Laxity which can be global laxity, or just anterior laxity of the dominant shoulder presenting in individuals with internal impingement occurring alone.

Anterior instability with apprehension or the feeling of subluxation when the arm is abducted and externally rotated.

Rotator cuff pathology can present as those with other rotator cuff diseases (other impingements, rotator cuff tears). Generally, younger patients and those who practice throwing sports are at much higher risk, and there should be a greater suspicion of internal impingement.

Some studies have found that internal impingement is the leading cause of rotator cuff dysfunction for sportspeople.

Clinical examination

Clinical history is vital for the proper diagnosis and management of internal impingement. However, as with external impingement, the history alone is not sufficient for a diagnosis, as many of the presenting symptoms are mercurial or non-reliable. The examination to assess shoulder dysfunction is summarized in Table-2.1.

TABLE-2.1: SUMMARY OF THE EXAMINATION TO ASSESS SHOULDER DYSFUNCTION	
Clinical Technique	**Findings**
Inspection for asymmetry	Affected joint may show wasting and lies lower than the contralateral side Non-regular scapular movement (scapulothoracicrhythm)
Palpation the shoulder joints	Tenderness along the joint line
Testing gross motor strength of the muscles of the shoulder	Weakness in the rotator cuff, serratus anterior, rhomboids and middle and lower trapezius muscles
Testing the mobility of surrounding joints	Reduced dorsal gleno-humeral glide and posterior capsule tightness
Testing for the flexibility of the cervical and thoracic spine and shoulder	Variable flexibility of each joint
Testing the range of movement of the gleno-humeral, scapulo-thoracic joints	ROM of GH rotation (internal and external) but 10 to 15 degrees

Clinical tests for the diagnosis of internal impingement include:

The posterior impingement sign assess the presence articular rotator cuff tears and posterior labral lesions. The test can be used to rule out posterior rotator cuff tears, as it has a specificity of 85% and a sensitivity of 75.5%.

The test is positive if it induces deep posterior shoulder pain when the arm is abducted (90° to 110°) and extended (10° to 15°) and fully externally rotated (98).

The relocation test

Jobe and colleagues (2000) suggested that the test is effective in diagnosing internal impingement. If posterior shoulder pain is alleviated by posteriorly-applied force to the proximal humerus.

These tests may not have a sufficient amount of empirical evidence to support their efficacy.

DIFFERENTIAL DIAGNOSIS OF EXTERNAL IMPINGEMENT INCLUDES:

Gleno-humeral arthritis which is characterized by osteophytes formation on the inferior humeral head.

Nerve palsy which presents with wasting of infraspinatus and supraspinatus. It can be diagnosed with MRI of the shoulder or EMG. It can be caused by space-occupying lesions.

Recurrent anterior or multi-directional gleno-humeral instability which can be diagnosed as impingement in the young and those with labral detachment. It is the positive apprehension sign, or a negative anesthetic injection test.

Cervical spondylosis (radiculitis)

Frozen shoulder (non outlet impingement) with tissue contractions can cause the head of humerus to translate when the shoulder is flexed resulting in impingement, even in the absence of acromion pathology.

Posterior capsule contracture with loss of internal rotation can present similarly to impingement.

AC joint arthritis can be excluded with negative anesthetic injection test.

Paralysis of the trapezius

Inter-articular pathology which presents with bony crepitus and significantly hindered passive movement. An AP or axillary X-ray may show arthritis.

Calcific tendinitis
Cuff tear arthropathy
Biceps tendonitis
Reflex sympathetic dystrophy
Thoracic outlet syndrome
Osacromiale

DIFFERENTIAL DIAGNOSIS OF INTERNAL IMPINGEMENT

It is necessary to remember that many of the clinical signs of internal impingement can occur in healthy patients; as such, the whole clinical picture is necessary. A doctor must take the following factors into consideration: age, occupation, fitness, disease severity and general wellbeing.

When a patient presents with symptoms and signs that do not a particular diagnosis, internal impingement syndrome need to be considered.

CHAPTER THREE: SHOULDER ANATOMY

The girdle of the shoulder consists of three bones (the clavicle, the scapula and the humerus) that make contact in three joints (sterno-clavicular, acromion-clavicular and gleno-humeral).

This conglomeration of three joints allows for a wider range of movement.

The gleno-humeral joint is most important as it forms a synovial articulation of the head of humerus and the glenoid. The glenoid space that the humerus articulates with is encircled by a fibro-cartilaginous labrum which deepens the joint, and increasing its stability.

The humeral head and the glenoid cavity are lined in hyaline cartilage which is thicker in the centre of the cavity and thinner around the edges. The whole gleno-humeral joint is surrounded by a fibrous capsule.

The rotator cuff consists of four muscles and their tendons which attach to the humerus and stabilizes the joint.

The subscapularis is present at the anterior of the joint and lying in the subscapularis fossa below the scapula. It inserts at the lesser tuberosity of the humerus and has fibers transverse humeral ligament which lie over the bicipital groove (Figure-3.1).

The supraspinatus (Figure-3.2) lies in the supraspinatus fossa above the scapula. It inserts at the greater tuberosity of the humerus.

The infraspinatus (Figure-3.3) lies posteriorly in the infraspinous fossa in the scapula. It is located just above the **teres minor muscle** (Figure-3.3) which is the fourth muscle of the rotator cuff, and both muscles insert at the greater tuberosity.

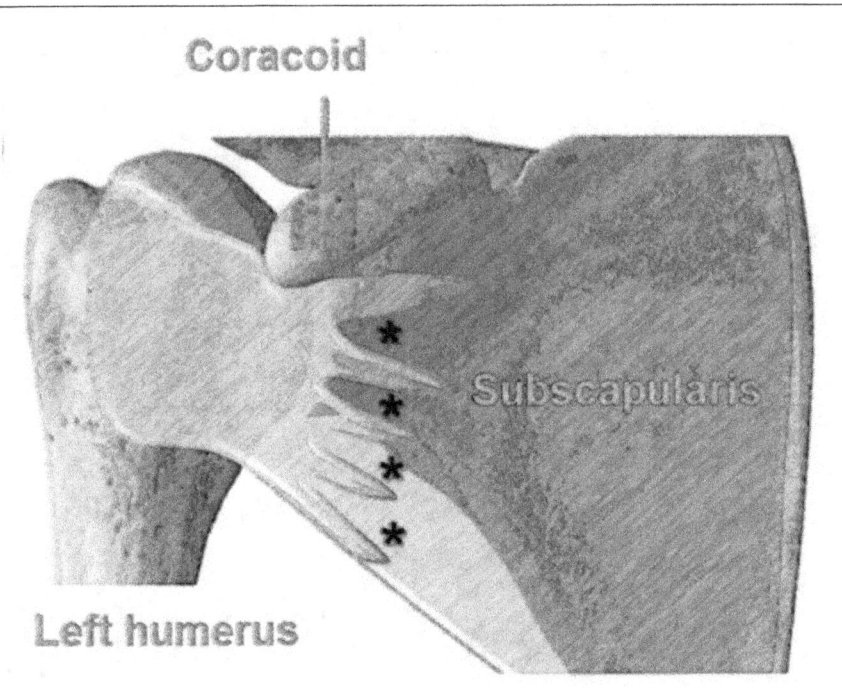

Figure-3.1: The subscapularis muscle originates at the subscapular fossa, runs superiorly and laterally below the coracoid, and anterior the gleno-humeral joint. The muscle inserts at the lesser tuberosity of the humerus. This muscle and tendinous fibers alternate to form the tendon (as represented by the asterisks)

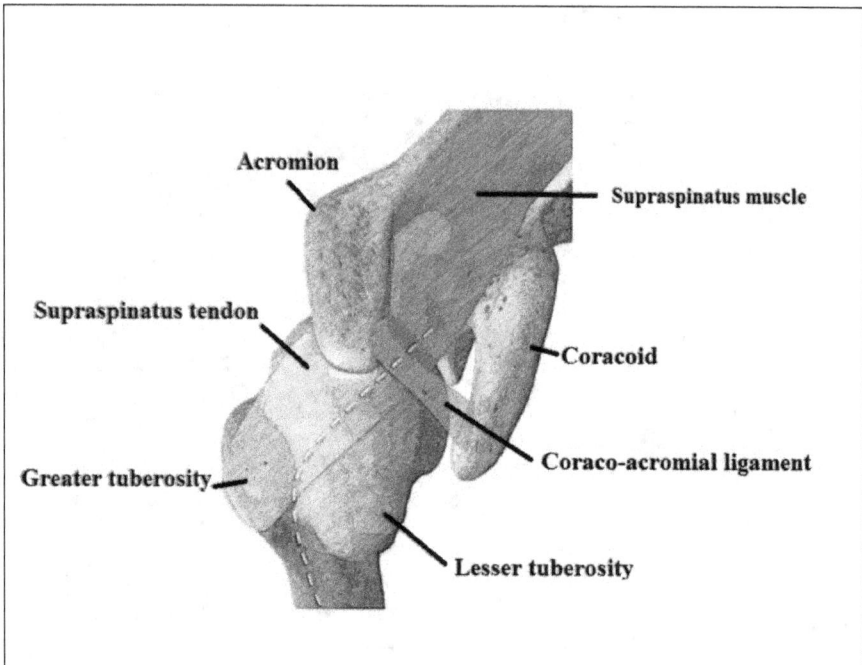

Figure-3.2: The supraspinatus muscle originates at the medial third of the supraspinous fossa and the homonymous fascia. It runs laterally posterior to the lateral clavicle, and inferior to the acromion and the coraco-acromial ligament. It inserts on the superior humeral greater tuberosity running along the long head of biceps tendon

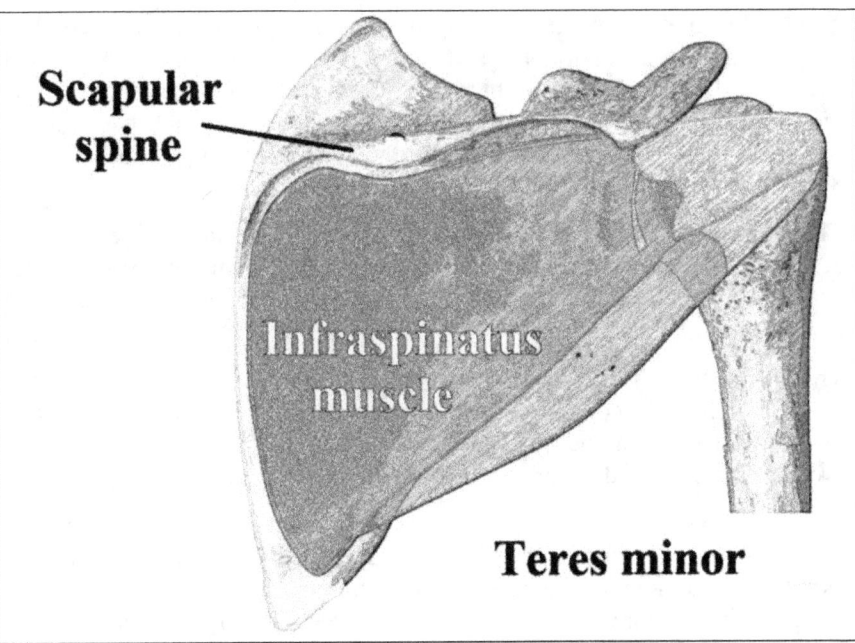

Figure-3.3: The infraspinatus muscle is a triangular muscle originating at the medial part of the fossa infraspinata and the infraspinous fascia. It continues a tendon laterally, running under the acromion, inserting on the lower facet of the greater tuberosity of the humerus. Teres minor is a long flat muscle originating at the fossa infraspinata, its tendon runs superiorly and laterally, inserting at the postero-inferior aspect of the humeral greater tuberosity.

The long head of biceps tendon (Figure-3.4) is the only tendon in the area which has a synovial sheath communicating with the gleno-humeral joint cavity. is not exactly part of the rotator cuff muscle, but it can be evaluated when the shoulder joint examined with an ultrasound.

The rotator interval houses the superior gleno-humeral ligament (medial or deep to long head of biceps tendon) and coraco-humeral ligament (superficial to long head of biceps tendon) .These ligaments create the biceps pulley, covering the long head of biceps tendon as it enters the bicipital groove; this further enhances the stability of the tendon (Figure-3.5).

The subacromial-subdeltoid bursa is a synovial space located beneath the acromion, between the superior supraspinatus tendon and the coraco-acromial arch (an arch consisting of the acromion, the coracoid and the coraco-acromial ligament).

The bursa extends in front of the bicipital groove and inwards to the coracoid where it continues as the subcoracoid bursa. The lateral and posterior margins of the bursa are less consistent, generally reaching the greater tuberosity of the humerus (Figure-3.6).

The acromion-clavicular joint; this is a diarthrodial synovial joint located between the medial acromion and the distal (convex) clavicle. The articular aspects of the join are separated by a fibro-cartilaginous disc and are surrounded by a fibrous capsule. This joint is stabilized by the following: the coraco-clavicular, coraco-acromial and acromio-clavicular ligaments.

A thorough knowledge of bone anatomy is vital in order to properly understand the anatomical positioning of the rotator cuff.

The greater tuberosity of the humerus consists of three facets (superior, middle and inferior) which attach to three of the rotator cuff tendons.

The supraspinatus tendon (20mm in width) attaches to the upper portion of the middle facet and the whole of the superior facet.

The infraspinatus (22mm in width) attaches to the middle facet, and has a 10mm overlap with the supraspinatus tendon.

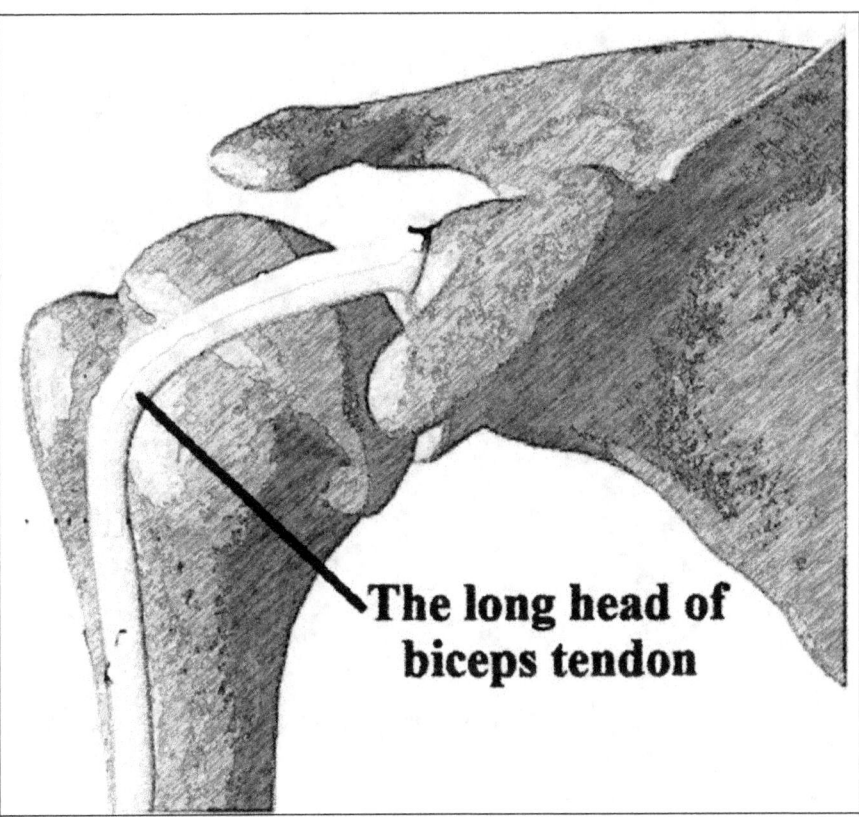

Figure-3.4: The long head of biceps tendon originates at the supra-glenoid tuberosity of the scapula and the glenoid labrum. The horizontal portion begins as a long and cylindrical tendon running into the shoulder joint cavity between the humeral head and the joint capsule. The angular portion runs downwards, between lesser and greater tuberosity. The vertical portion runs into the bicipital groove of the anterior aspect of the humerus covered by an extension of the synovial capsule

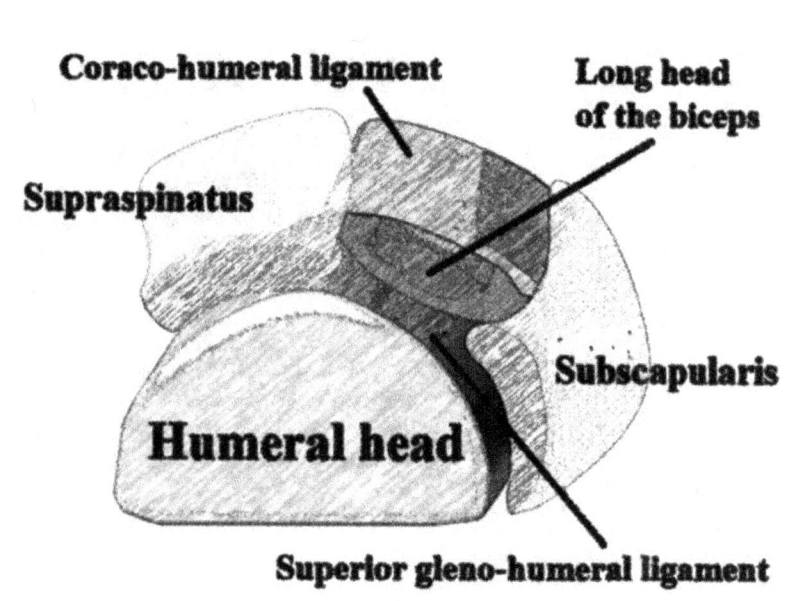

Figure-3.5: The rotator interval is a free space between the subscapularis and supraspinatus tendons. The coraco-humeral ligament is superficial to the long head of the biceps tendon; the superior gleno-humeral ligament is deep to it. These two structures, together with the tendinous portion of the subscapularis, form the long head of biceps tendon pulley

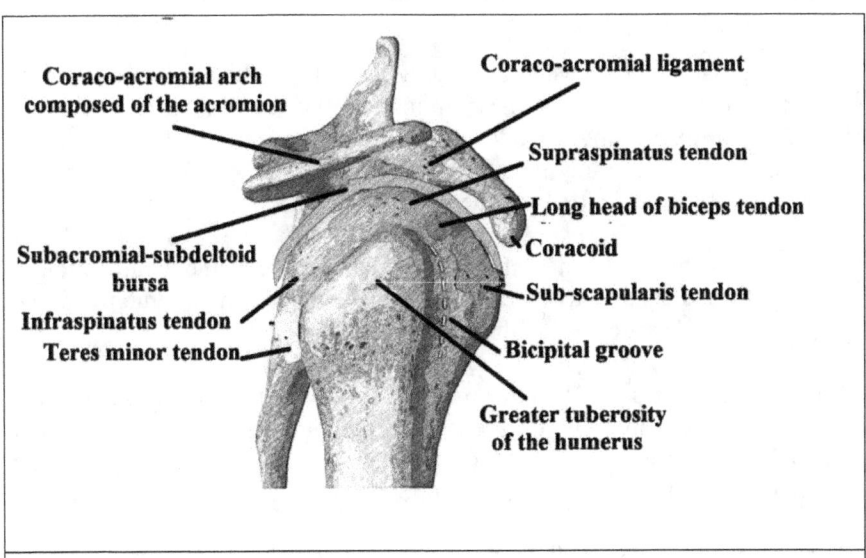

Figure-3.6: structures of the shoulder (Lateral view)

The teres minor tendon attaches to the inferior facet, at the posterior portion of the tuberosity (see Figure-3.6), the sulcus neighboring the tuberosity (1.5-2mm in width), the whole head of humerus is layered with articular cartilage. Lying beyond the sulcus is the insertion of the supraspinatus tendon. The place where this tendon thickens at the insertion is called the supraspinatus footprint.

CHAPTER FOUR

IMAGING DIAGNOSTIC MODALITES: PLAIN FILMS (X-RAYS, RADIOGRAPHS)

Plain x-ray is used first when evaluating shoulder pathology because of its low cost and minimal invasiveness. In many instances, Plain x-ray is all that is needed for diagnosing shoulder pathology, and even if further imaging is necessary, the initial x-ray must be properly assessed in order to determine which the next investigation to order is.

The complex shoulder joint commonly demands more than one projection in to properly understand the local anatomy. Generally, a minimum of two perpendicular planes covering the area are produced.

The scapula creates a 45° angle with the thorax in the frontal plane. This means that the planes of the gleno-humeral joint and the thorax are not parallel to one another, and that the gleno-humeral joint will be in an oblique position when a traditional AP (antero-posterior) radiograph is obtained.

Plain AP x-rays taken while the shoulder is internally or externally rotated are insufficient for diagnosing most shoulder pathologies including calcification of the cuff tendons. Rotating the humerus does not adjust the position of the scapula, and a minimum of two projections are necessary; AP and lateral projections are the traditional options.

It is necessary to capture both the AP and the 'actual AP' (40° posterior oblique, in order to capture the real AP of the gleno-humeral joint, and to obtain an axillary view and a modified Y scapula view (or the 'outlet view'). This is generally enough for conditions such as arthritis, instability, trauma and impingement. However, further views may be necessary for certain shoulder pathologies.

The antero-posterior projection (Figure-4.1A) is the core projection in x-ray radiography. This projection requires two plain radiographs: one whilst the arm is rotated externally and one whilst it is rotated internally.

Due to the 40° antero-lateral position of the gleno-humeral joint, the head of humerus and the glenoid overlap in these images (Figure-4.1A).

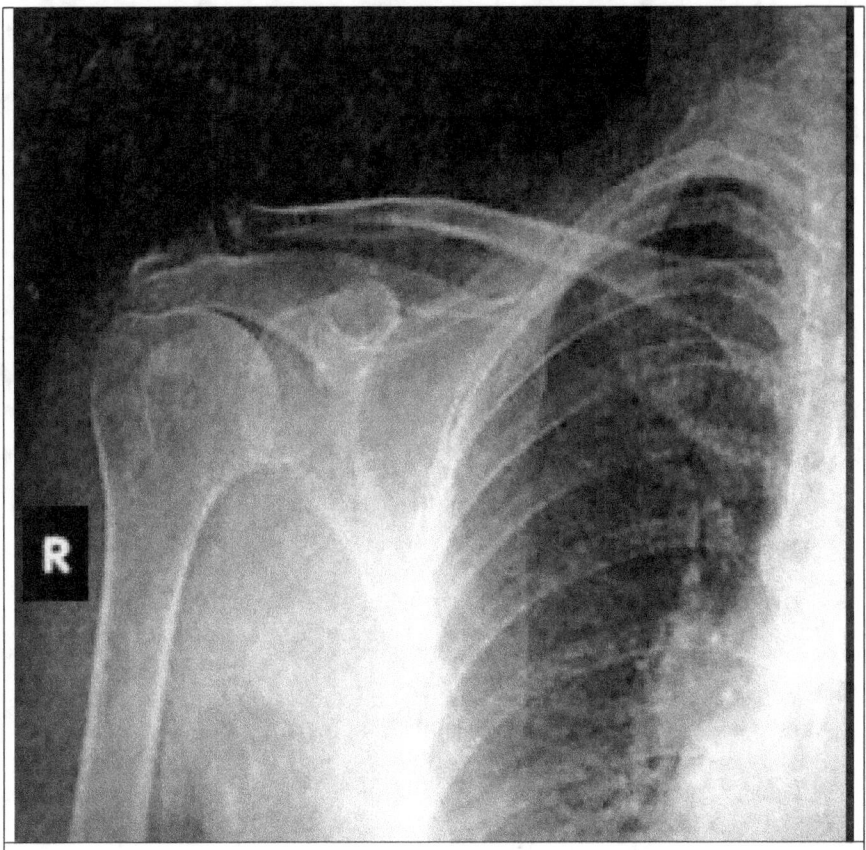

Figure-4.1A: Antero-posterior (AP) projection with the arm in a neutral position.

The traditional AP view displays the AC and gleno-humeral joints, and the distal clavicle, and can be used in the evaluation of the following features:

The relationship between the glenoid cavity and the humerus. An 'empty glenoid' suggests a posterior dislocation: the overlap will be reduced or will disappear entirely.

The relationship between the acromion and the distal portion of the clavicle.

The epiphysis of the proximal humerus, and its any irregularities.

The tracks for the tendons of supraspinatus and infraspinatus, and the presence of calcifications.

The inferior acromion and the presence of osteophytes.

The postero-lateral head of humerus. A Hill-Sachs lesion may be revealed through internal rotation; this is a compression fracture that is caused by recurrent anterior dislocations.

The gap between the humerus and the acromion; normally this space is 7-14mm in length. A reduced gap suggests a rotator cuff tear. An AP view can be taken with and without stress in order to elucidate an AC injury. The stress is induced by asking the patient to carry 5kg in each hand in order to force traction in the arm. A 'step sign' is seen in the AC space if there is 3rd degree AC trauma.

A Grashey projection used to obtain an actual **AP of the gleno-humeral joint** (not normally obtainable due to the position of the scapula).

In order to obtain a true AP image, the film should be performed by firing X-rays at 45° to the gleno-humeral joint (from the medial to the lateral).

The Grashey projection allows the physician to look at the glenoid distinctly from the head of humerus (Figure-4.1B). An overlap in this projection suggests a dislocation anteriorly or posteriorly.

The actual AP is also useful in spotting gleno-humeral arthritis, coracoid/glenoid/humeral fractures and posterior instability of the joint.

The Grashey projection can also assess the location of the head of humerus (in relation to the glenoid), the presence of AC arthritis, rotator cuff calcification and acromion osteophytes.

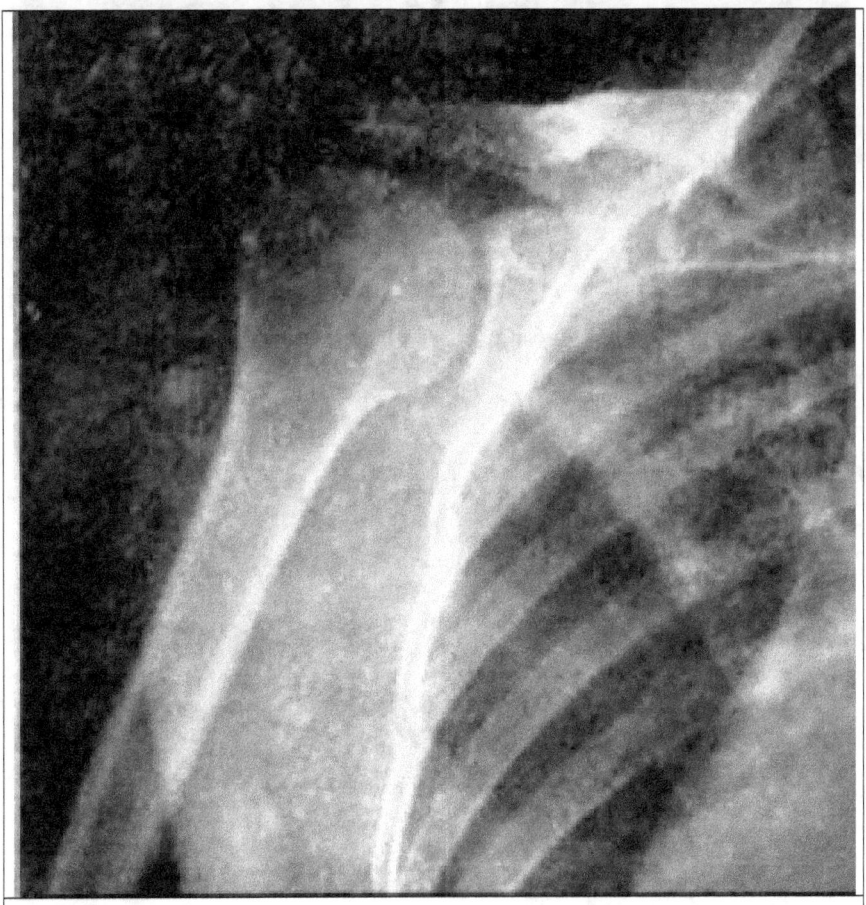

Figure-4.1B: Actual AP (Grashey) projection

The axillary projection demonstrates the relative positions of the humeral head and the glenoid, and allows for the diagnosis of dislocation (Figure-4.1C).

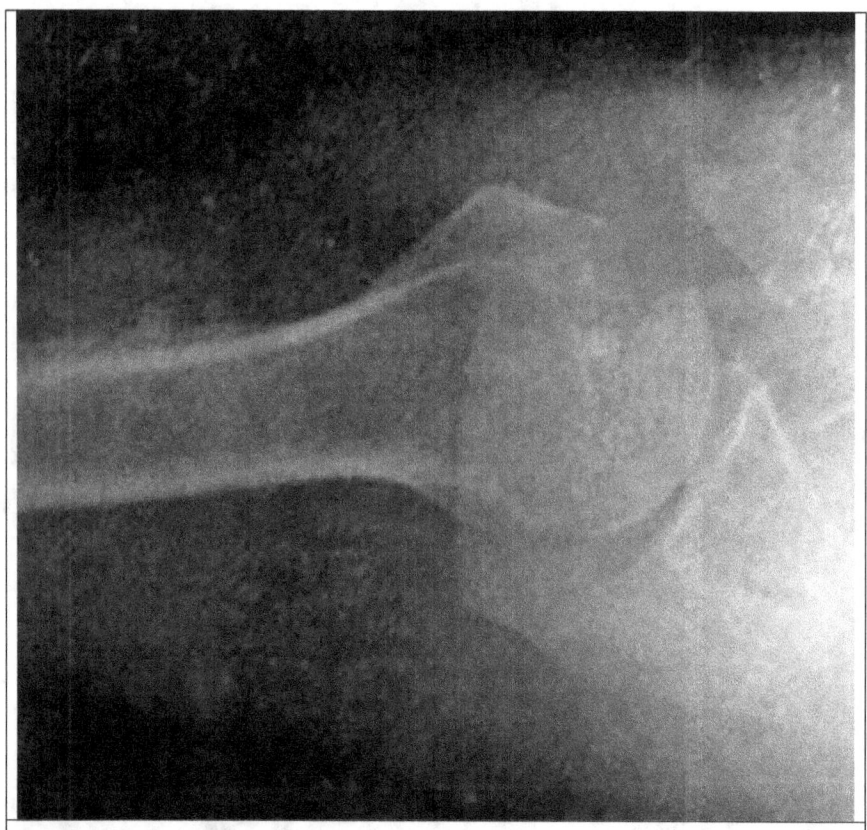

Figure-4.1C: Axillary projection

The radiograph must be obtained whilst the arm is abducted by 70-90°, and whilst the patient is supine or standing.

The X-rays are fired at the axilla inferior to superior, with the film above the shoulder. This projection is particularly suitable for demonstrating the space between the glenoid and humeral head.

Reduced of the gleno-humeral joint space suggests cartilage loss in the joint.

The axillary projection can also clearly show subluxation, dislocation, compression fractures of the humerus (such as Hill-Sachs lesions) and fractures of the glenoid rim.

The axillary view also allows for detailed assessment of glenoid erosion, AC abnormalities, coracoid/acromial fractures and osacromiale. However, trauma may mean that patients cannot abduct their arm sufficiently; in such cases, an axillary projection may not be obtainable.

Outlet" (modified scapular Y) projection is used to visualize a cross-section of the outlet of the supraspinatus towards the arm. It shows details of the acromion, the space beneath it and its inferior surface (Figure-4.1D).

The inferior surface is especially important to examine, as it has significant consequences for surgery. An outlet projection radiograph, in combination with a sagittal oblique cross-section MRI, is vital for accurately guiding an acromioplasty (a core component of rotator cuff operations).

The radiograph is obtained whilst the patient standing in front of a wall at an anterior oblique angle of 60°, with the shoulder in contact with the cassette.

The X-rays are then fired at a cranio-caudal angle of 15-30°. This positioning is an altered version of the scapular Y projection, in which the cranio-caudal angle is 0-10°. An outlet projection is taken in order to create a film with the following features: an overlap of the coraco-acromial curve and the curve of the scapula and spine (on the sagittal plane) (Figure-4.2A, B); a profile of the inferior acromion to aid in surgery.

The scapular Y projection (a basis for the outlet radiography), is otherwise known as the scapulo-lateral radiograph, tangential lateral radiograph, Y lateral radiograph or trans-scapular radiograph. These forms are often abbreviated to 'Y view'. A Y view radiograph is taken whilst the arm is medially rotated and externally supported; as such, in acute injury this is an easier position to induce than for the lateral axillary radiograph.

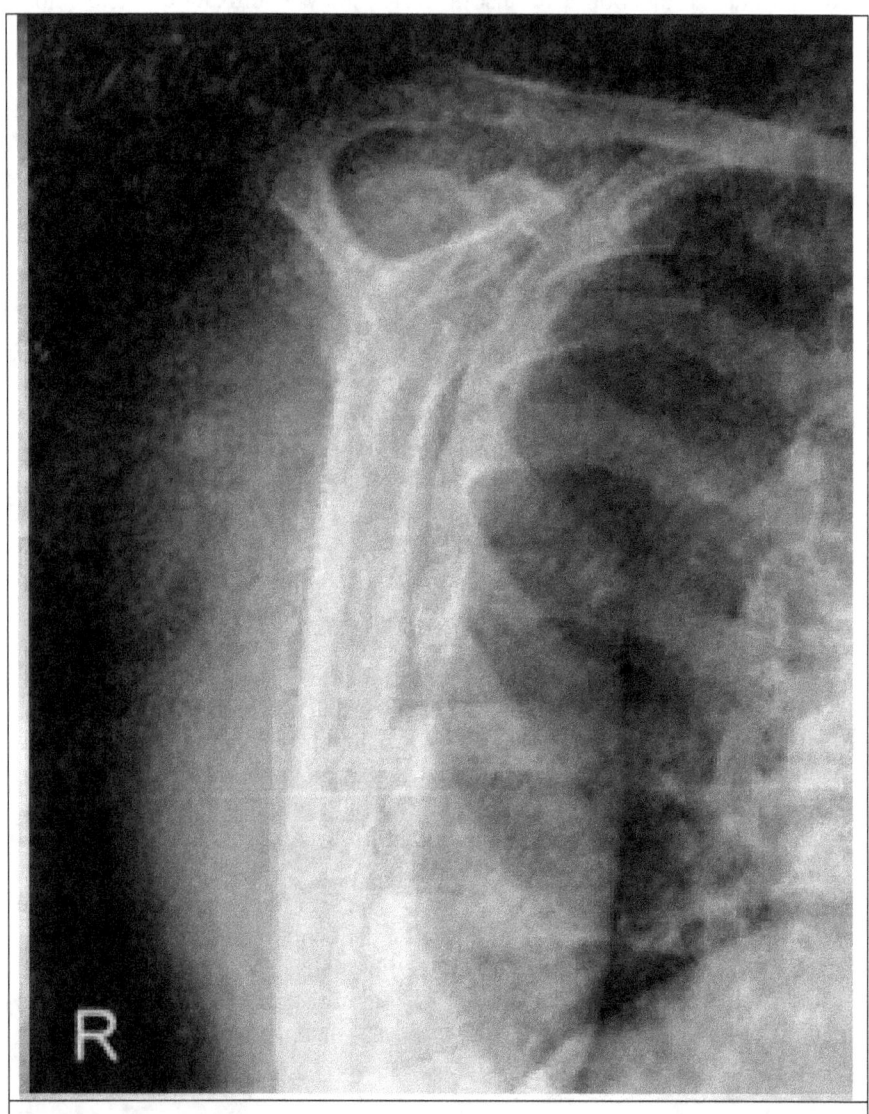

Figure-4.1D: Outlet projection

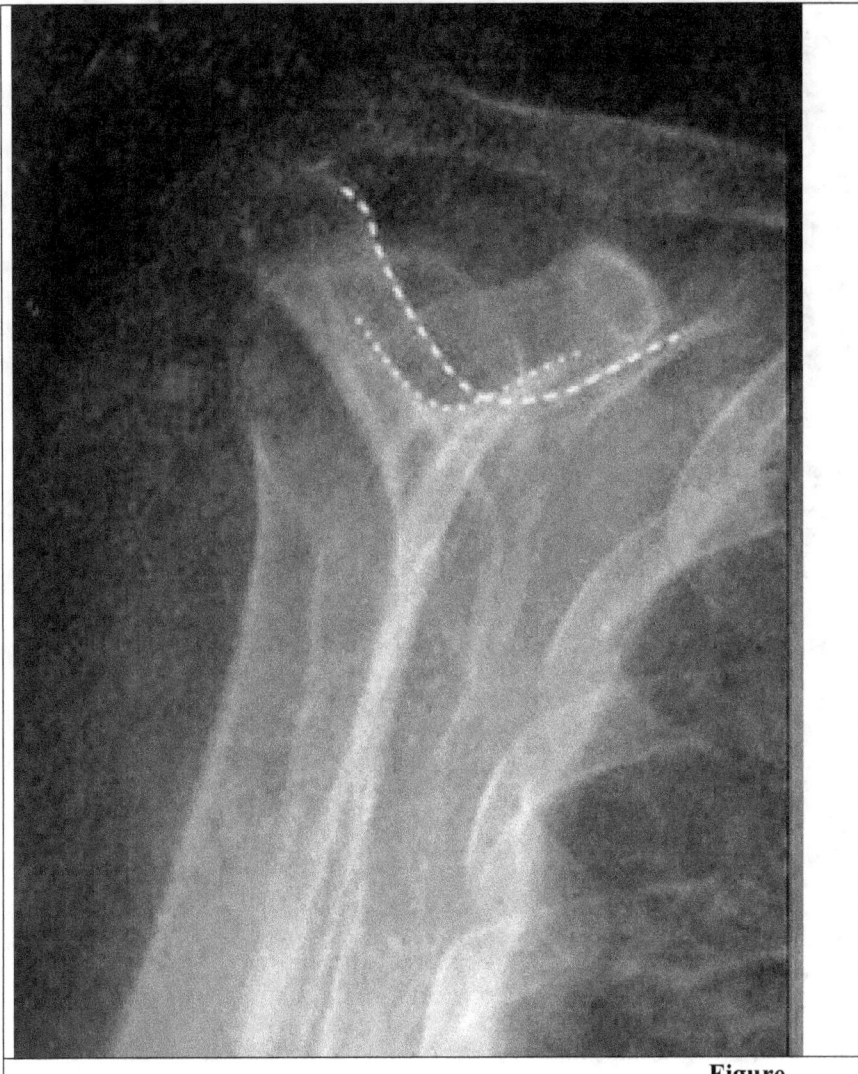

Figure-4.2A: Acceptable example for a shoulder outlet projection. Coraco-acromial arch (dashed line) does not overlap with the arch of the scapular body and spine (dotted line)

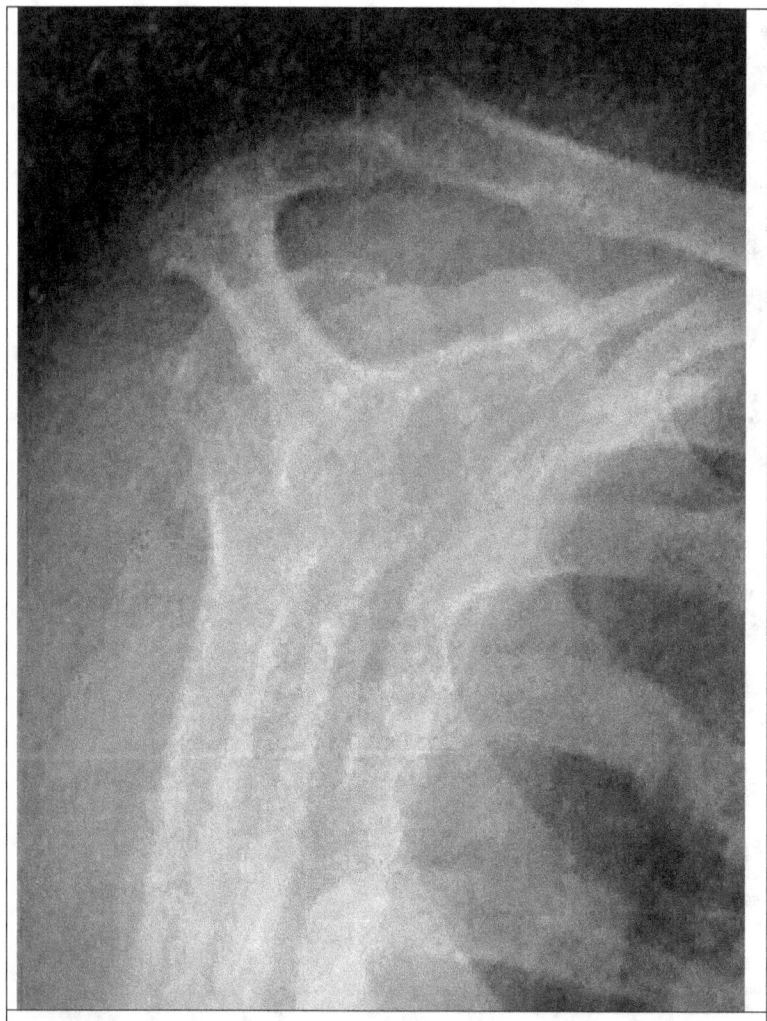

Figure-4.2B: Suboptimal example for a shoulder outlet projection. Coraco-acromial arch and the arch of the scapular body and spine overlap with each other, which is not optimal

A Y view projection shows the lateral aspect of the gleno-humeral joint, with the scapula creating the letter 'Y'. This Y is formed by the coracoid process in the anterior and the scapular spine posteriorly (forming the arms of the Y), whilst the body of the scapula forms the stalk of the Y. Where the three limbs of the Y meet, the glenoid fossa is positioned. When appropriately obtained, a Y view radiograph will show an overlap of the lateral and medial borders of the scapula.

The Y view projection is particularly suitable visualizing the relationship between the head of humerus and the glenoid fossa (in the sagittal oblique plane). When the head of humerus is anteriorly displaced relative to the glenoid fossa, there is likely an anterior dislocation. Likewise, if the humeral head is posteriorly displaced in relation to the glenoid fossa, it is probably a posterior dislocation.

Y view projections are not able to reveal fractures of the glenoid rim, but are able to detect fractures of the greater humeral tubercle. Whilst it is possible to more clearly visualize Hill-Sachs lesions (in comparison to axillary radiographs), the real specialty of the scapulo-lateral projection is its ability to detect dislocation and proximal humeral fractures.

The combination of the outlet projection with the true AP and lateral axillary projections, three distinct views of the joint (perpendicular to one another) are available. This provides the clearest picture of the joint to physicians, and is therefore the ideal combination (Table-4.1 and Figure-4.1).

TABLE 4.1: RECOMMENDED SERIES OF STANDARD RADIOGRAPHS FOR THE SHOULDER
AP projection in neutral shoulder position An AP of the shoulder, with no rotation of the arm.
Actual AP projection Grashey projection. Arm is closer to and 45° posterior oblique to the cassette.
Axillary projection Patient supine or standing, arm abducted 70-90°, X-rays fired caudo-cranially at the cassette placed over the shoulder.
Outlet" projection Modified scapular Y view. Arm closer to cassette and is 60° anterior oblique to the cassette. X-rays fired 15-30° caudo-cranially.

CHAPTER FIVE
IMAGING DIAGNOSTIC MODALITES: ULTRASONOGRAPHY

Ultrasonography is frequently used to assess the shoulder joint and its pathologies including tendinosis, tendon tears, bursitis, instability, entrapment and synovial joint issues.

In the hand of expert operator, an ultrasound can be as effective as an MRI.

Ultrasound scans are cheap, easily available, and has the ability to produce images in high resolution and does not use ionizing radiation like some other imaging modalities.

Ultrasonography allows dynamic assessment of the musculoskeletal system in the area, giving it another advantage over other modalities.

In the hand of expert, ultrasonography can diagnose rotator cuff tears at 100% (complete tears) or 91% (partial tears) accuracy. However, this accuracy is highly dependent on the operator and the conditions of the environment and machine.

When assessing a joint using ultrasound, a protocol (see Table-5.1) including a checklist of core structures is necessary.

Using this tool is vital for a comprehensive and effective ultrasound scan.

Studies reported that many patients' symptoms do to not accurately correlate with the location of the lesion, and a focused ultrasound exam may not detect up on all elements of the pathology.

It is vital to have a thorough understanding of the anatomy of the area, as most of the accuracy of ultrasound exams are dependent on the quality of the technique of the operator. A good operator needs to know bone anatomy and tendon orientation comprehensively. It is also important to note the limitations of ultrasonography technique, such as anisotropy.

TABLE-5.1: ULTRASOUND PROTOCOL
Step No. 1 Biceps brachii tendon, long head
Step No. 2 Subscapularis and biceps brachii tendon, subluxation/dislocation
Step No. 3 Supraspinatus and rotator interval
Step No. 4 Acromio-clavicular joint, subacromial-subdeltoid bursa, and dynamic evaluation for subacromial impingement
Step No. 5 Infraspinatus, teres minor, and posterior labrum

ULTRASOUND EXAMINATION TECHNIQUE

When starting the examination, a short history can help guide the procedure to follow. For instance, pain radiating to the elbow that wakes a patient at night is indicative of rotator cuff pathology. It is also important to ask about trauma, infection and any masses. Also, note the age, as patients over 40 are more like to have a cuff tear, whilst those under 40 are more likely to have labral pathology.

From start to finish, a shoulder ultrasound can last just 10 minutes, even being less than 5 minutes long if the shoulder is healthy. However, a comprehensive assessment, using the protocol, is necessary for an adequate ultrasound scan.

Step 1: Biceps brachii tendon, long head.

The patient places their hand palm face up on their lap. The transducer is positioned in the axial plane over the anterior shoulder (Figure-5.1A).

The bicipital groove is located using its unique contours, with the surface of the humerus appearing hyperechoic with posterior acoustic shadowing. The long head of biceps tendon lies within this groove, visible in the short axis (Figure-5.1B). Due to the deep natures of the biceps tendon, the tendon itself might appear artifactually hypoechoic due to anisotropy (Figure-5.1C).

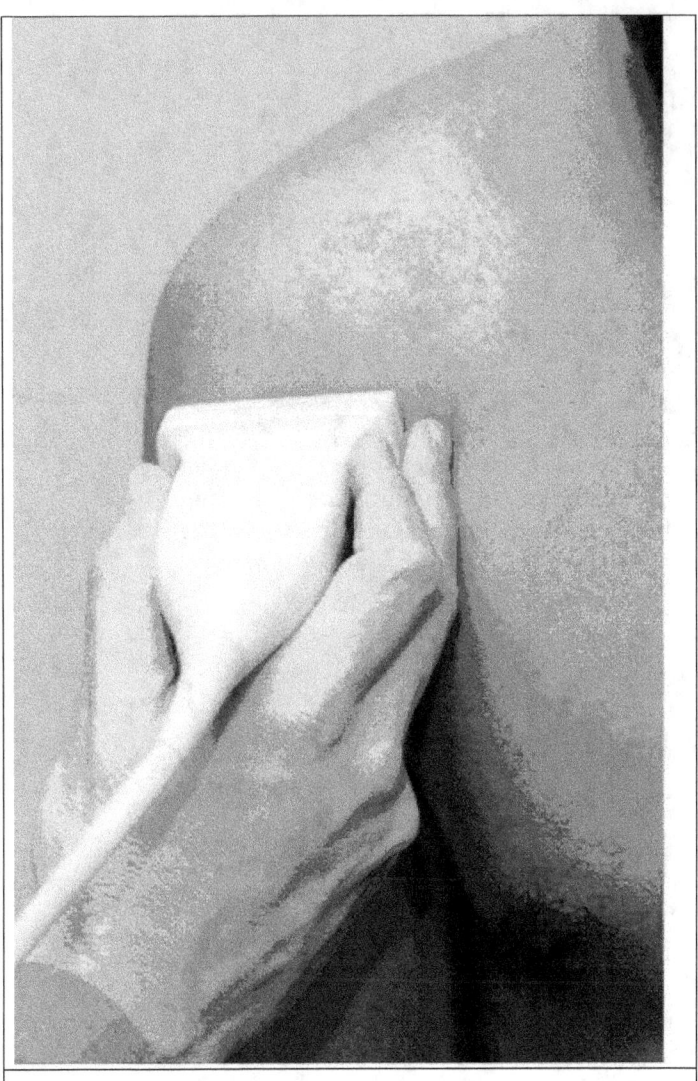

Figure-5.1A: Long head of the biceps brachii tendon (short axis). Transducer placement.

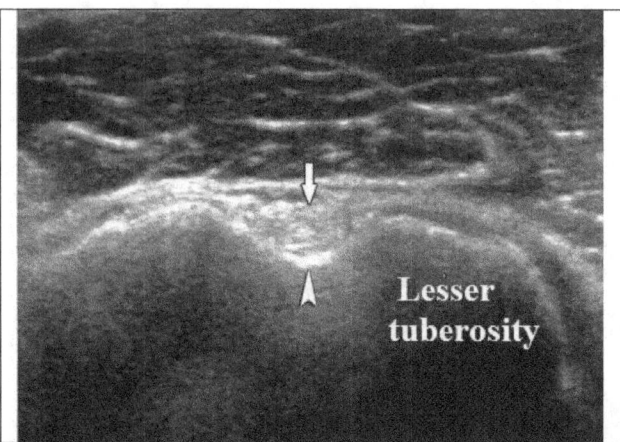

Figure-5.1B: Long head of the biceps brachii tendon (short axis). Corresponding ultrasound image showing long head of the biceps brachii tendon (arrow) in the bicipital groove (arrowhead); Right side of image is medial

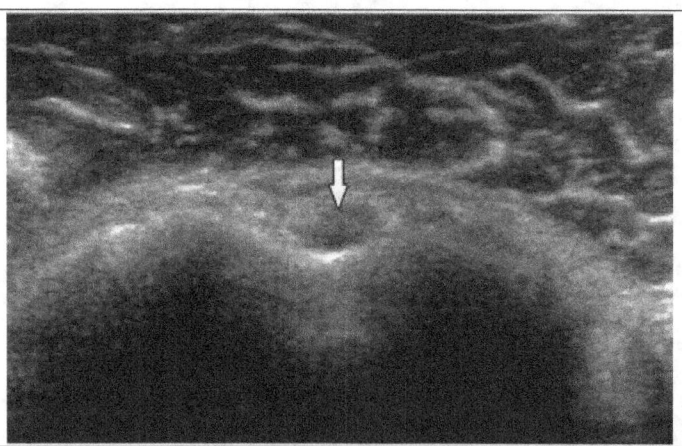

Figure-5.1C: Long head of the biceps brachii tendon (short axis). Ultrasound image shows the hypoechoic appearance of the tendon (arrow) due to anisotropy

The tendon is assessed for any malformations such as tears or tendinosis. Joint fluid suggests tenosynovitis. Only a miniscule amount of fluid would be expected in a healthy adult.

Step 2: Subscapularis and biceps tendon subluxation/dislocation

Following on from the previous procedure, the transducer remains over the anterior shoulder (axial plane) and the bicipital groove is located (Figure-5.1A). The subscapularis tendon can be visualized in the long axis, running anteriorly towards the lesser tuberosity, art factually hyperechoic due to anisotropy (Figure-5.2A). The patient then rotates their shoulder externally (Figure-5.2B). This rotates the lesser tuberosity laterally; the subscapularis (inferior to the coracoid) is pulsed laterally: this reduces anisotropy, as the tendon fibers are perpendicular to the ultrasound beam (Figure-5.2B). The operator must be sure to visualize the superior subscapularis, as this is the location of most tears in the tendon.

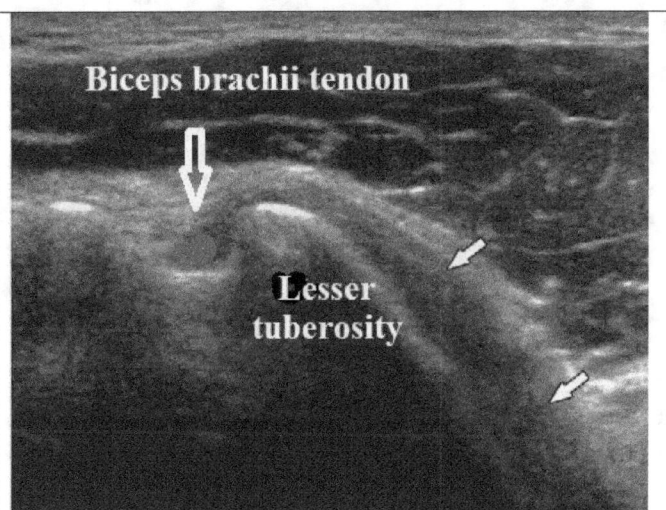

Figure-5.2A: Subscapularis tendon (long axis). Centered over lesser tuberosity, ultrasound image shows subscapularis tendon (arrows) artif-actually hypoechoic from anisotropy; Right side of image is medial

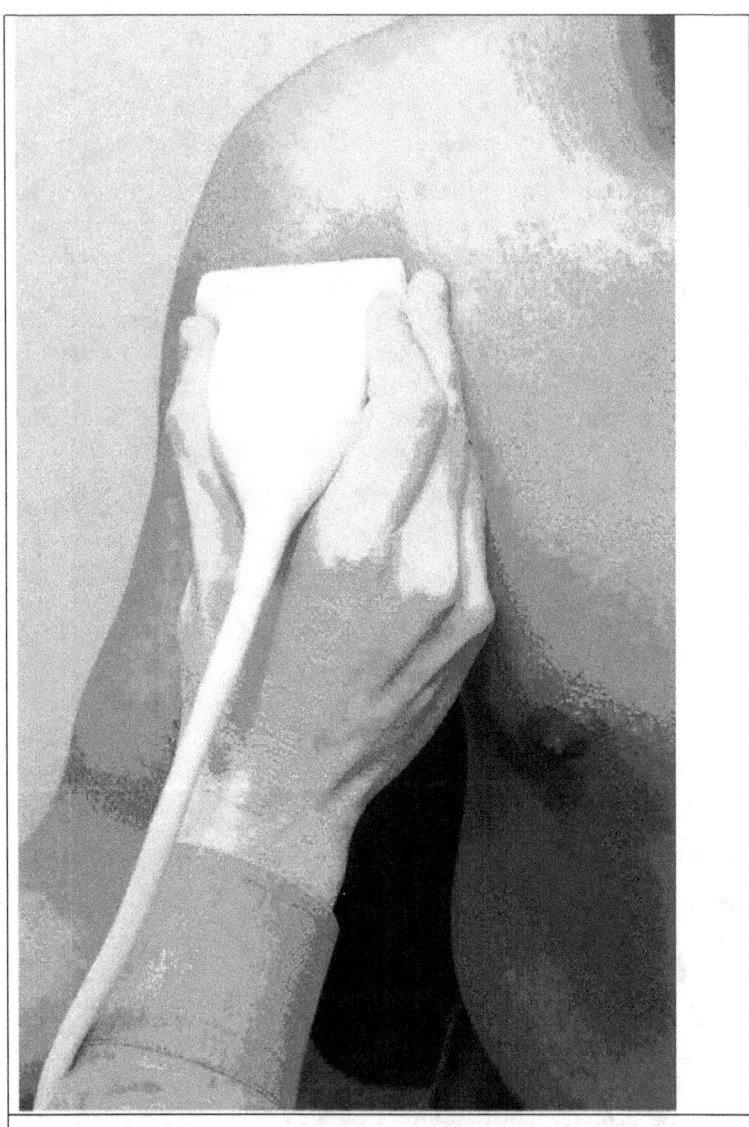

Figure-5.2B: Subscapularis tendon (long axis).Transducer placement with shoulder externally rotated

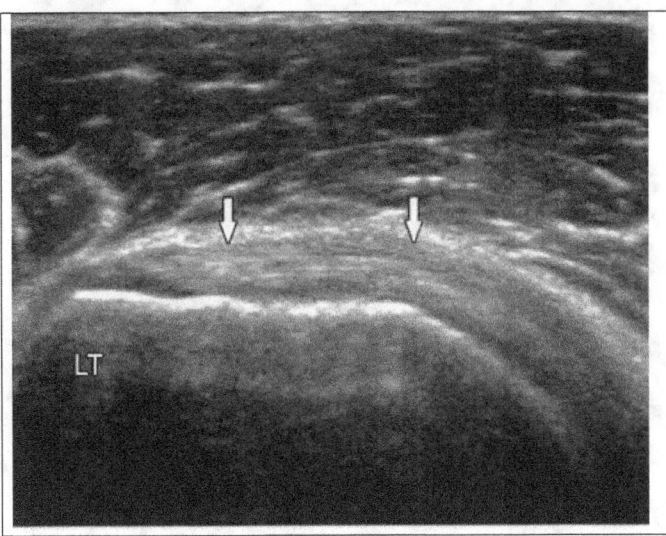

Figure-5.2C: Corresponding ultrasound image showing hyperechoic and fibrillar subscapularis tendon (arrows)

After this, the transducer is rotated 90° (Figure-5.3A) in order to locate the tendon in the short axis (Figure-5.3B). The transducer is rotated another 90° in the long axis, and laterally located to the bicipital groove to ensure that the long head of biceps tendon is properly located in this groove. If the tendon is partially outside this space, this is subluxation; if it is completely outside this space, this is dislocation. Figure-5.3B shows ultrasound image with hypoechoic tendon bundles due to anisotropy (arrowheads).

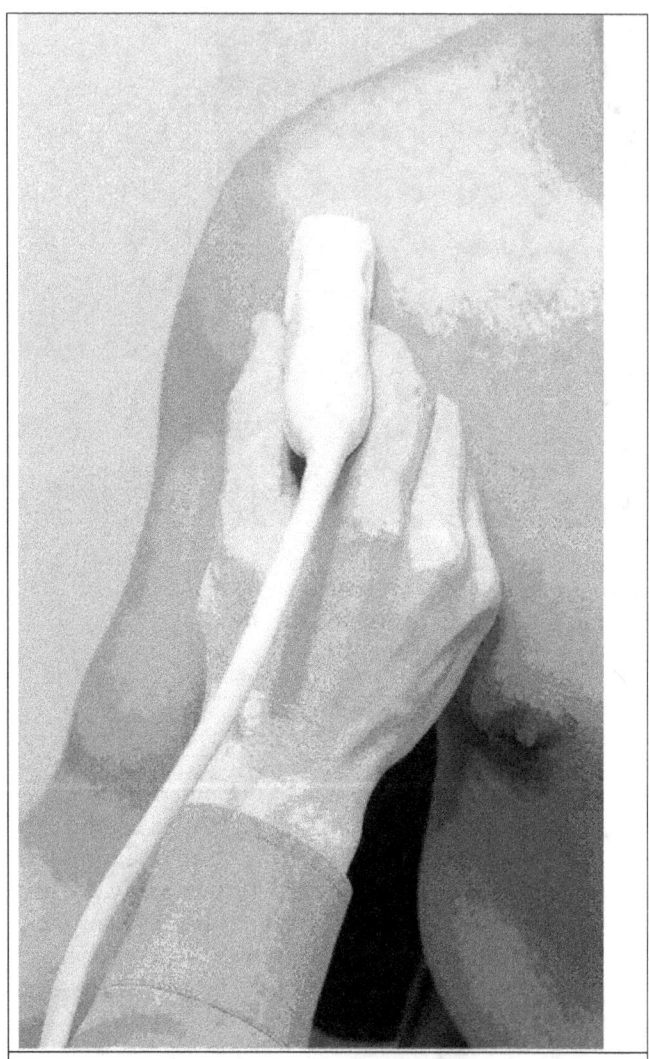

Figure-5.3A:Subscapularis tendon (short axis).Transducer placement, shoulder externally rotated

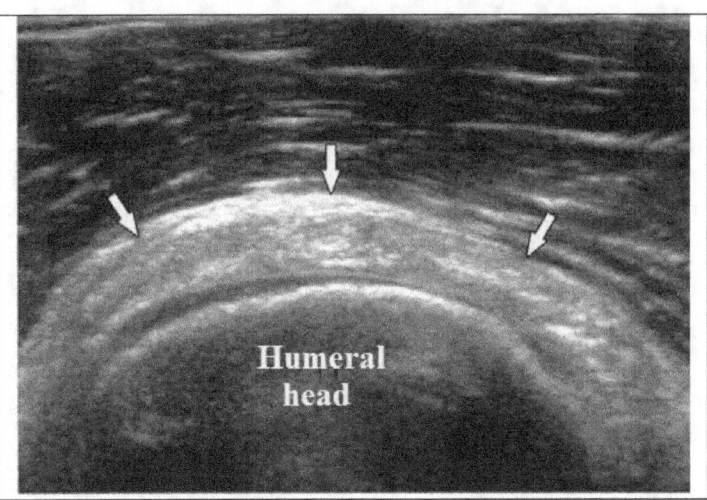

Figure-5.3B: Subscapularis tendon (short axis). Corresponding ultrasound image shows hyperechoic and fibrillar subscapularis tendon (arrows). Right side of image is inferior

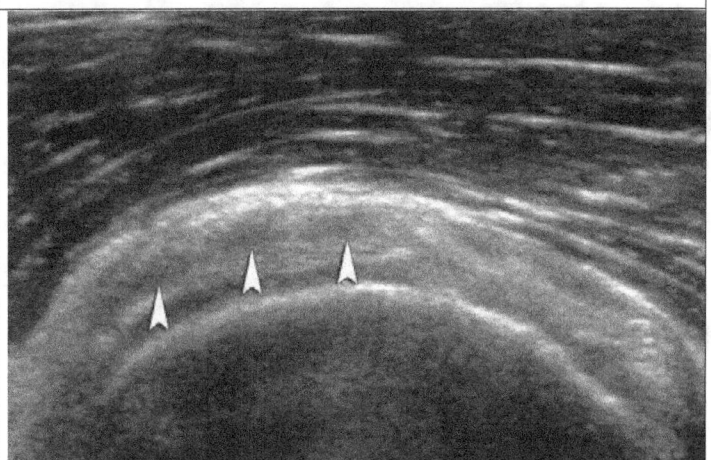

Figure-5.3C: Subscapularis tendon (short axis). ultrasound image shows hypoechoic tendon bundles due to anisotropy (arrowheads)

Step 3: Supraspinatus and rotator interval

Proper imaging of the supraspinatus enables recognition of the greater tuberosity and its bony landmarks. The greater tuberosity shifts as the shoulder is moved.

The traditional position used in ultrasound scans was the crass position with the dorsal ipsilateral hand is placed behind the back, in the crass position. This internally rotates and hyperextends the joint, pulling out the supraspinatus tendon from below the acromion.

In the Crass position, the greater tuberosity becomes anterior; the transducer is placed in the sagittal plane over the shoulder, providing a long axis view of supraspinatus.

The modified Crass position improves upon this position; the patient's ipsilateral hand is positioned on the ipsilateral buttock (Figure-5.4A), providing clear visualization without discomforting the patient.

The modified crass position allows for clear visualization of the supraspinatus in the long axis (Figure-5.4B). A long axis view demonstrates features of all the anatomic surfaces of the tendon (greater tuberosity, bursal, intra-articular), thereby allowing a detailed assessment of a tendon tear (complete, intra-substance, bursal or articular).

Figure-5.4C shows ultrasound image over rotator interval showing long head of biceps brachii tendon (arrows). Figure-5.4D shows ultrasound image over middle facet of greater tuberosity showing flattening of the greater tuberosity (arrowheads) in relation to the humeral head.

It is important to remember two things when assessing supraspinatus:

First, the whole width of the greater tuberosity must be assessed (front to back) by moving the transducer 2-2.5cm over the area.

Second, proper evaluation of the rotator interval is necessary, as many cuff tears occur here; this is why the crass position is so important.

An ultrasound of the tendon should begin anterior to the rotator interval and long head of biceps tendon; this makes sure that the whole anterior portion of the tendon is included.

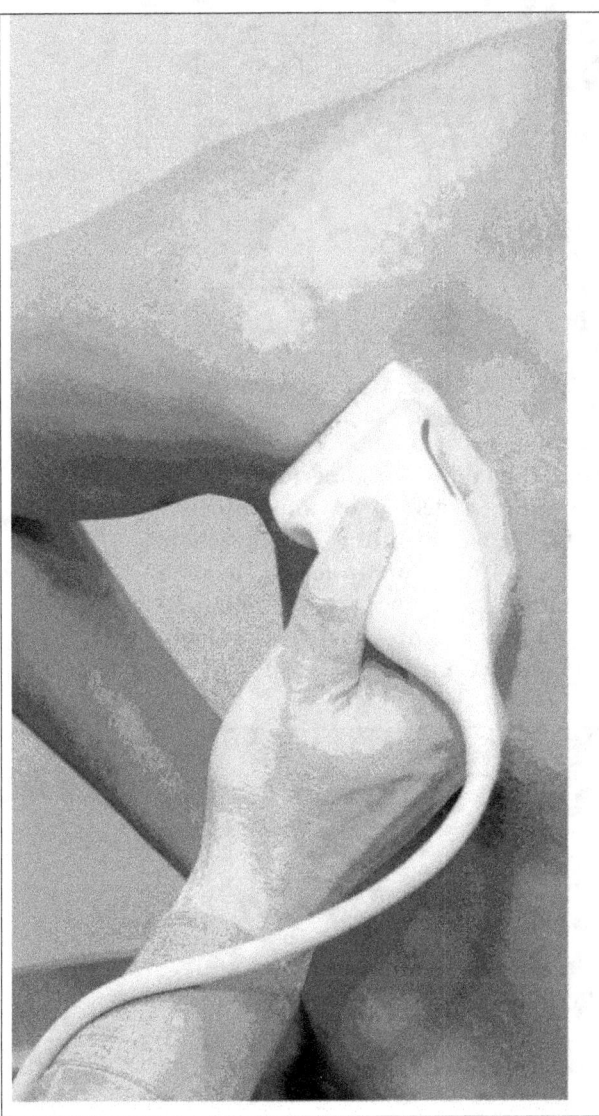

Figure-5.4A:Supraspinatus tendon (long axis).Transducer placement, shoulder in modified crass position

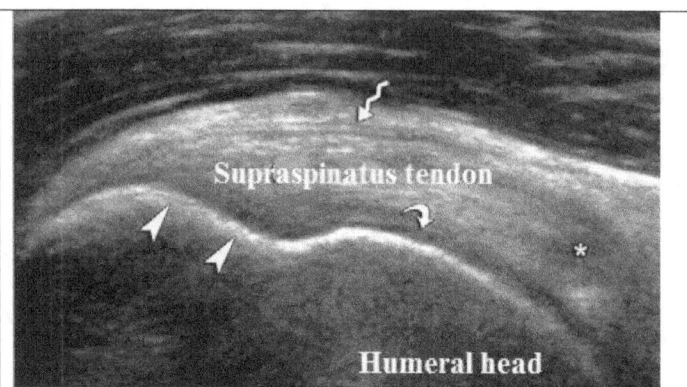

Figure-5.4B: Supraspinatus tendon (long axis). Corresponding ultrasound image over superior facet of greater tuberosity, showing hyperechoic and fibrillar supraspinatus tendon, demonstrating hypoechoic anisotropy (*). The superior facet (arrowheads), hyaline articular cartilage (curved arrow) and collapsed hypoechoic subacromial-subdeltoid bursa (squiggly arrow); The right side of image is medial

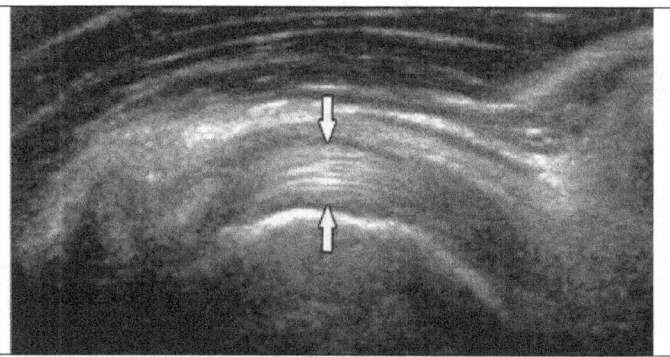

Figure-5.4C: Supraspinatus tendon (long axis). Ultrasound image over rotator interval showing long head of biceps brachii tendon (arrows)

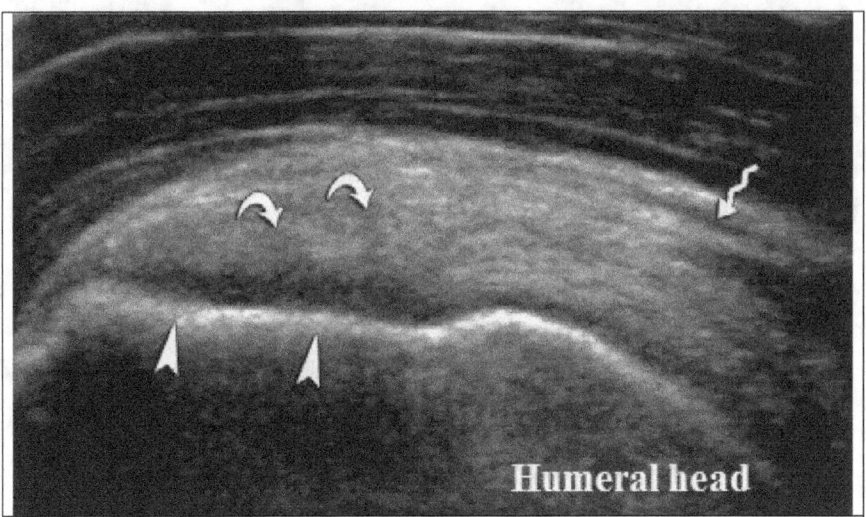

Figure-5.4D: Supraspinatus tendon (long axis). Ultrasound image over middle facet of greater tuberosity showing flattening of the greater tuberosity (arrowheads) in relation to the humeral head. The hypoechoic lines (curved arrows) from anisotropy at the junction of the supraspinatus and infraspinatus

A healthy supraspinatus tendon should be fibrillar in natural, with a hyperechoic and convex superior surface. As the fibers curve away from the US beam, the transducer should be constantly repositioned in order to minimize anisotropy.

After assessment of the supraspinatus in the long axis, the transducer is turned 90° in order to assess the short axis (Figure-5.5A). The transducer begins at the articular humeral head; a smooth and round echogenic surface (humeral head) and shallow layer of hypoechoicity that covers the rotator cuff (hyaline cartilage) indicates the positioning is correct. This is in the short axis of supraspinatus, 90° perpendicular to the long axis (Figure-5.5B).

It is vital that the rotator interval is correctly located (at the medial cuff) in order to locate the anterior supraspinatus. In the rotator interval itself, the long head of biceps is visible in the short axis, between the subscapularis and supraspinatus tendons. There will be a thin hyperechoic line (coraco-humeral ligament) lying superficial to the long head of biceps, with this ligament being a component of the pulley of biceps. In this pulley is the thin hyperechoic line that is the superior gleno-humeral ligament, lying medial to the long head of biceps.

After the intra-articular section of the supraspinatus tendon has been assessed, the ultrasound transducer is gradually moved to the greater tuberosity.

Once the articular surface ends, the supraspinatus footprint will become visible at the level of the greater tuberosity, allowing for visualization of the superior and middle facets of the tuberosity. These facets must be identified to properly localize pathology in the infraspinatus (middle facet) or supraspinatus (superior middle facet).

Moving the transducer distally will show the tendons tapering and ending over the facets.

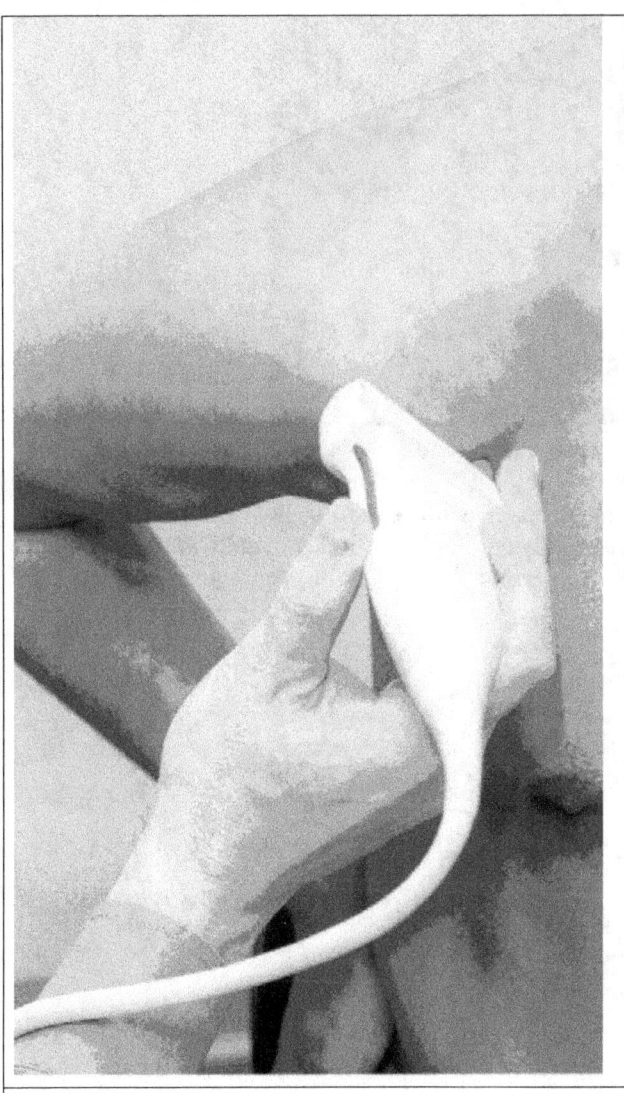

Figure-5.5A:Supraspinatus tendon (short axis).Transducer placement with shoulder in modified crass position

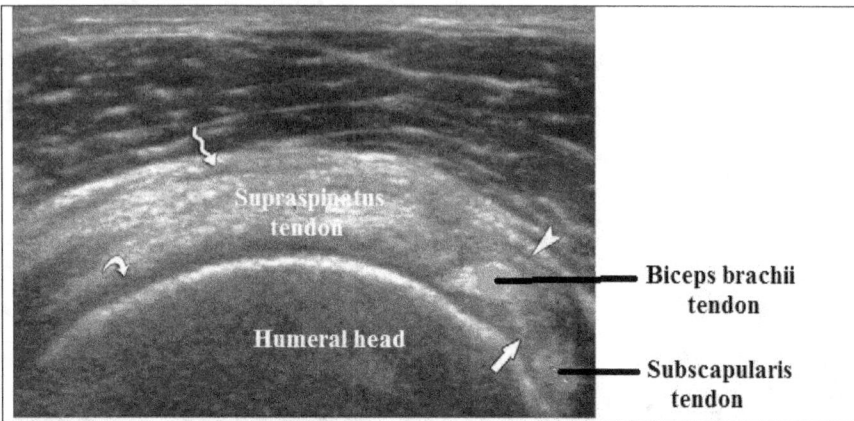

Figure-5.5B: Supraspinatus tendon (short axis).Corresponding ultrasound image over humeral head shows hyperechoic and fibrillar supraspinatus tendon. Biceps brachii tendon in the rotator interval with superficial coraco-humeral ligament (arrowhead) and medial superior gleno-humeral ligament (arrow).The right side of image is anterior

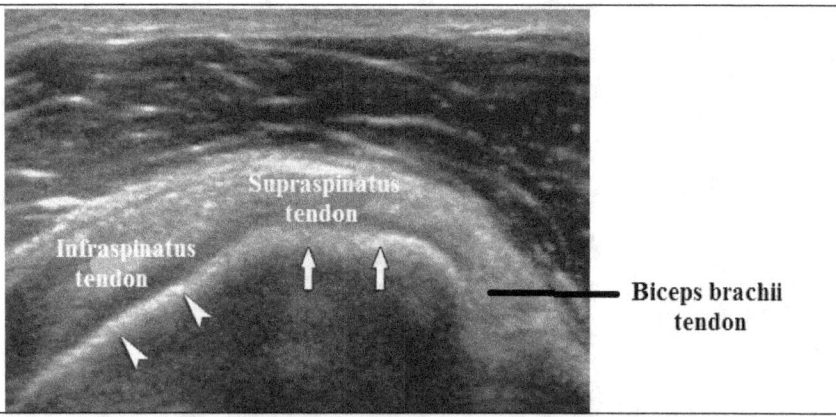

Figure-5.5C: Supraspinatus tendon (short axis). Ultrasound image distal to articular surface over greater tuberosity facets shows supraspinatus tendon adjacent to superior facet (arrows), and infraspinatus tendon adjacent to middle facet of greater tuberosity (arrowheads). The right side of image is anterior. Subscapularis tendon; hyaline cartilage (curved arrow); subacromial-sub-deltoid bursae (squiggly arrow)

Step 4: Acromio-clavicular joint, subacromial-subdeltoid bursa, and dynamic evaluation for subacromial Impingement

To identify the AC joint, the examiner needs to palpate laterally along the clavicle, until reaching the acromion. The transducer is placed along the coronal plane of the body, over the point (Figure-5.6A).

Another method involves the patient placing their palms up on their lap, with the transducer placed along the transverse plane over the frontal shoulder (in order to find the bicipital groove).The transducer is moved superiorly, allowing for visualization of the unique structures of the AC joint superior and proximal to the cuff and humeral head (Figure-5.6B).

The AC joint is then assessed for narrowing, widening, offset or bone irregularity. In the case of widening (or if AC disruption is suspected), dynamic evaluation is necessary to identify alignment changes.

Whilst evaluating the AC joint in the long axis (in relation to the clavicle), the patient must place their ipsilateral hand on the contralateral shoulder. This position allows a clinician to visualize unusual widening or offset, or bone contact of the clavicle and acromion; these features may be causing symptoms.

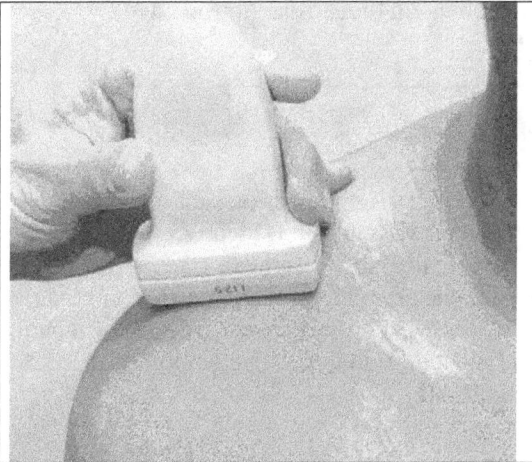

Figure-5.6A: Acromio-clavicular joint. Transducer placement over superior aspect of the shoulder

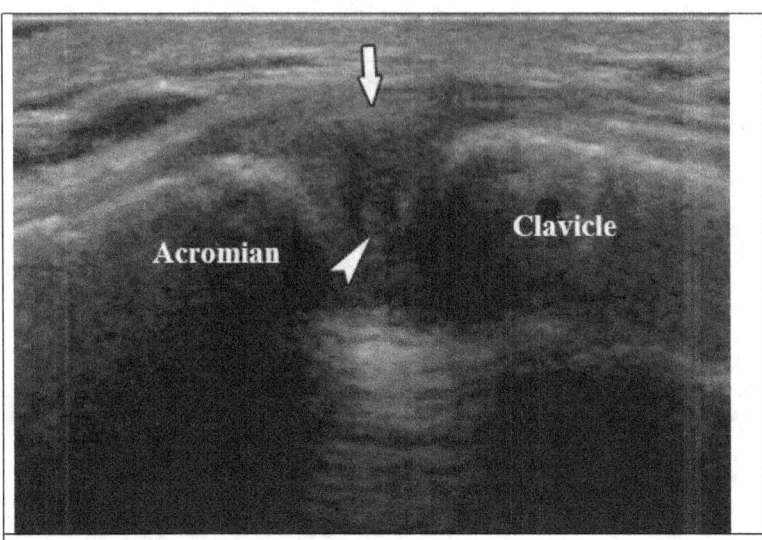

Figure-5.6B: Acromio-clavicular joint. Corresponding ultrasound image showing acromio-clavicular joint (arrow) with hyperechoic bone contours of the distal clavicle and acromion. There is echogenic fibro-cartilage disc (arrowhead). The left side of image is lateral

Dynamic assessment is used to look for impingement subacromially. The transducer is laterally moved to the lateral acromion (Figure-5.7A). Once the bony features of the greater tuberosity and acromion can be visualized (Figure-5.7B), the patient elevates the arm (Figure-5.7C). This can be done passively first, then actively. During active movement, the supraspinatus tendon and subacromial-subdeltoid bursa should move smoothly to below the acromion, out of sight (Figure-5.7D).

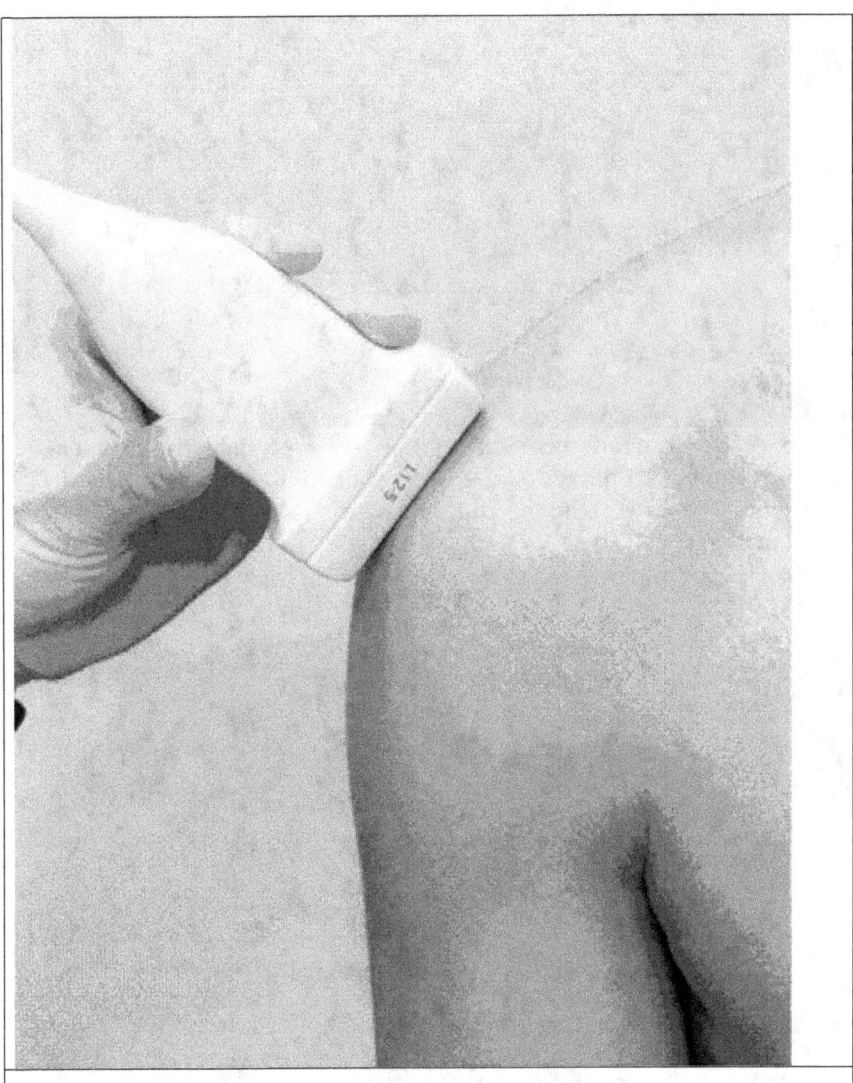

Figure-5.7A: Dynamic assessment for subacromial impingement. Transducer placement over supero-lateral aspect of shoulder in neutral position

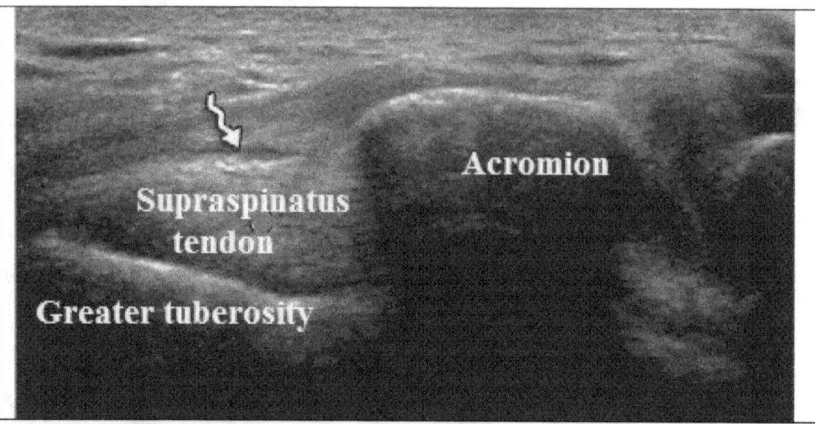

Figure-5.7B: Dynamic assessment for subacromial impingement. Corresponding US image shows acromion and greater tuberosity with supraspinatus tendon and collapsed subacromial-subdeltoid bursa (arrow)

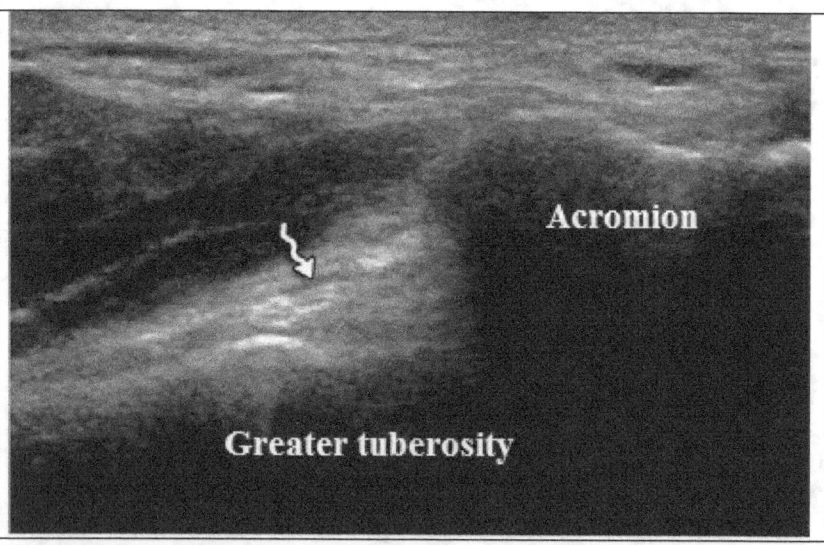

Figure-5.7C: Dynamic assessment for subacromial impingement. Ultrasound image showing the acromion, greater tuberosity and a normal collapsed subacromial-subdeltoid bursa (arrow). The left side of images is lateral

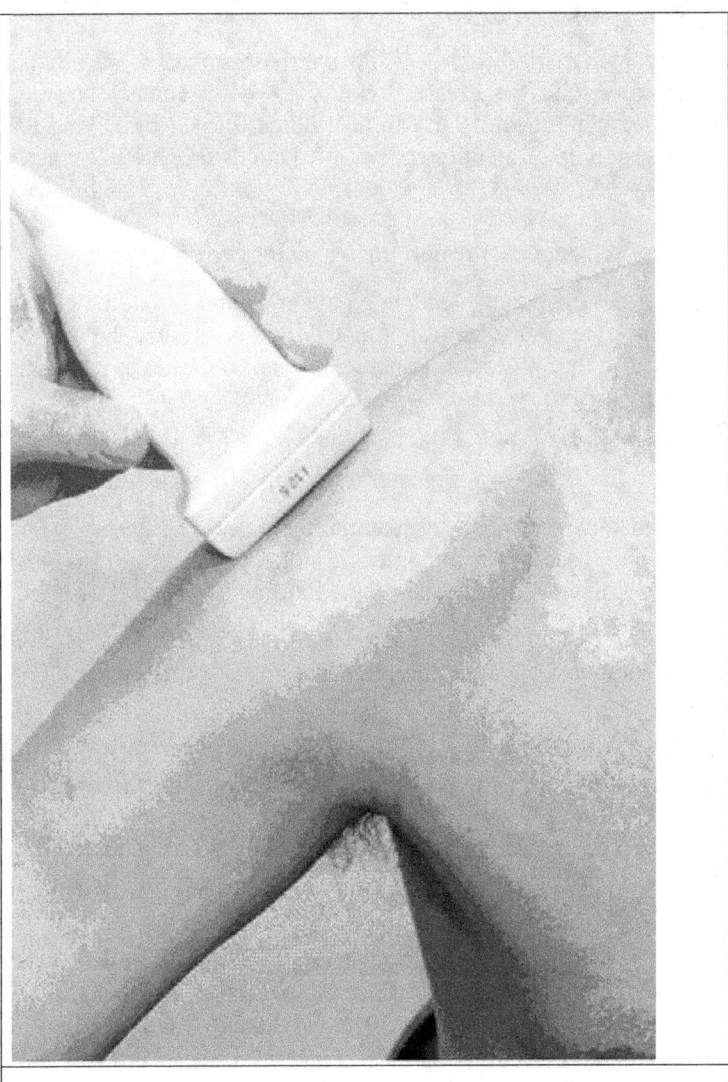

Figure-5.7D: Dynamic assessment for subacromial impingement. Transducer placement following abduction of the shoulder

Subacromial impingement may be indicated by the pooling of bursal fluid (at the lateral acromion) or by the snapping of bursal tissue.

Impingement may also be indicated by the interposition of supraspinatus between the acromion and the greater tuberosity, or by contact between those two bones. Dynamic evaluation can also be performed by having the patient raise their arm antero-laterally whilst their hand is pronated.

Step 5: Infraspinatus, teres minor and posterior labrum

In order to assess the infraspinatus tendon, a patient's hand should be placed palm up in the lap. The transducer should then be positioned below the scapular spine, over the posterior shoulder in an oblique axial plane (mirroring the scapular spine position) (Figure-5.8A).

This allows the operator to visualize the long axis of the infraspinatus tendon at its insertion point (at the posterior greater tuberosity) (Figure-5.8B).

By moving the transducer towards the scapula, the posterior labrum can be assessed (labral tears), as can the spinoglenoid notch (paralabral cysts) and the posterior gleno-humeral joint recess (joint fluid and synovitis) (Figure-5.8C).

The transducer is rotated 90° (Figure-5.9A) in order to see the tendon along its short axis (Figure-5.9B).

Sometimes acromial shadowing can make seeing the distal infraspinatus tricky; in cases like this, have the patient move their hand to the opposite shoulder. This position will pull the tendon to the anterior, allowing identification. However, by internally rotating the joint like this, the tendon becomes curved in appearance as it comes around the humerus; before, it was straight.

It is also necessary to look for lipo-degeneration and wasting of the infraspinatus muscle, as if this occurs in the presence of a tear it carries a poorer surgical prognosis for the patient. The transducer should be moved medially, covering the musculo-tendinous junction of the infraspinatus (short axis) (Figure-5.9C).

The echogenicity and size of the muscle at the junction should be compared with teres minor.

In a healthy adult, the muscle should be twice the size of teres minor, and have similar hypoechoicity (Figure-5.9D). If the is an increased echogenicity, lipo-degeneration is likely; a reduced size is indicative of atrophy. This positioning also allows for evaluation of teres minor at its insertion point.

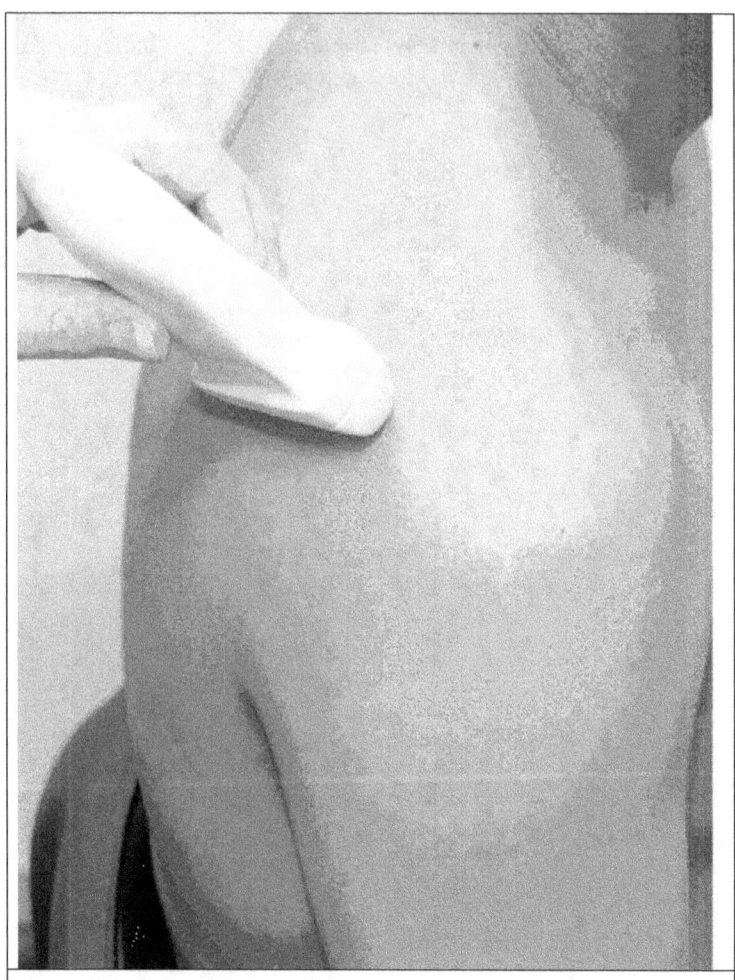

Figure-5.8A: Infraspinatus tendon (long axis), posterior gleno-humeral joint, and spinoglenoid notch. Transducer placement over posterior aspect of the shoulder in neutral position

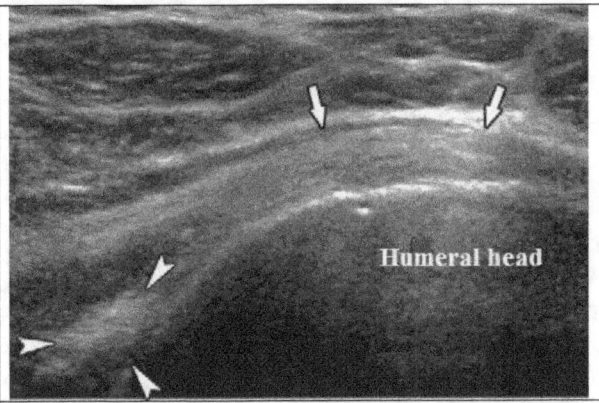

Figure-5.8B: Corresponding ultrasound image displaying contours of the humeral head (H) with neighboring infraspinatus tendon (arrows) and glenoid labrum (arrowheads)

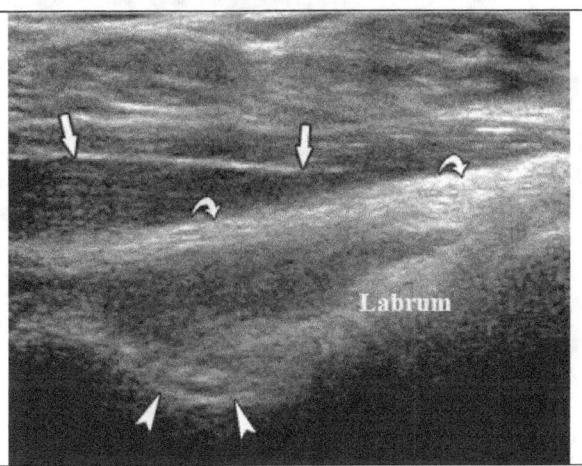

Figure-5.8C: Infraspinatus tendon (long axis), posterior gleno-humeral joint, and spinoglenoid notch. US image medial to b shows spinoglenoid notch (arrowheads) of scapula with neighboring suprascapular vessels. Note infraspinatus musculo-tendinous junction (straight arrows) and central tendon (curved arrows). The left side of image is medial

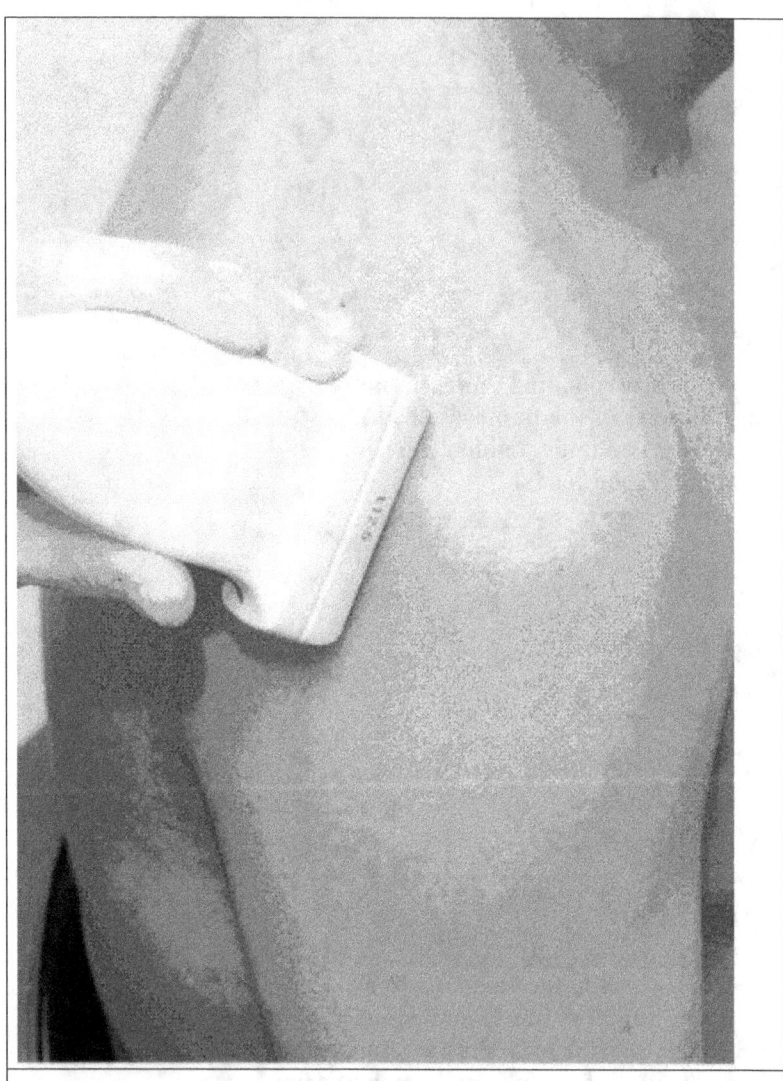

Figure-5.9A:Infraspinatus and teres minor (short axis).Transducer placement over posterior aspect of the shoulder in neutral position

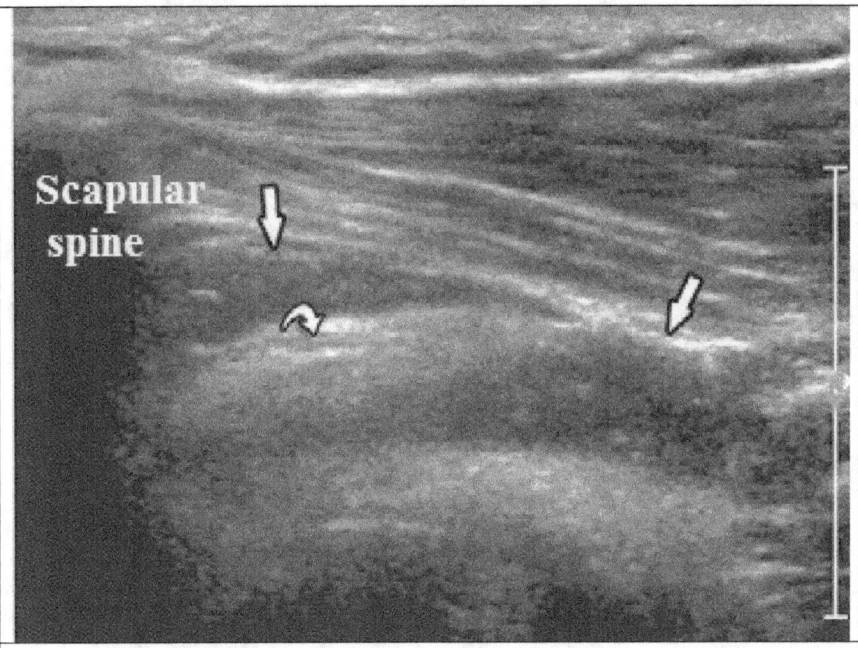

Figure-5.9B: Infraspinatus and teres minor (short axis). Corresponding ultrasound image shows infraspinatus (straight arrows) and central tendon (curved arrow). S =. Left side of image is superior

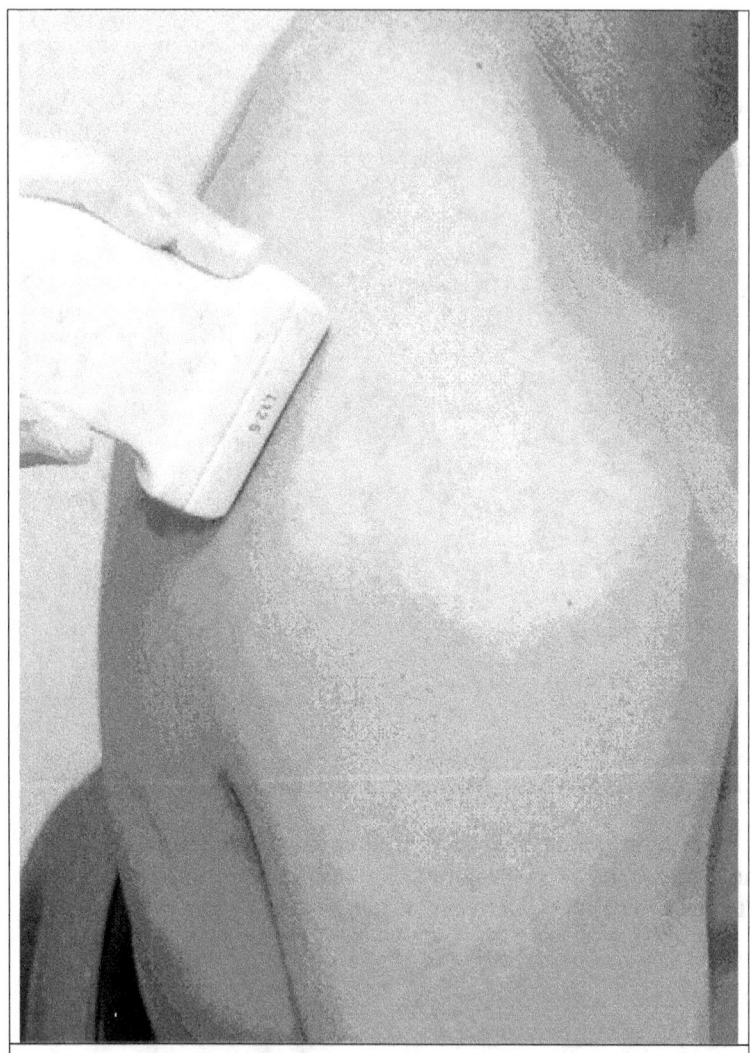

Figure-5.9C: Infraspinatus and teres minor (short axis). The transducer should be moved medially, covering the musculo-tendinous junction of the infraspinatus (short axis)

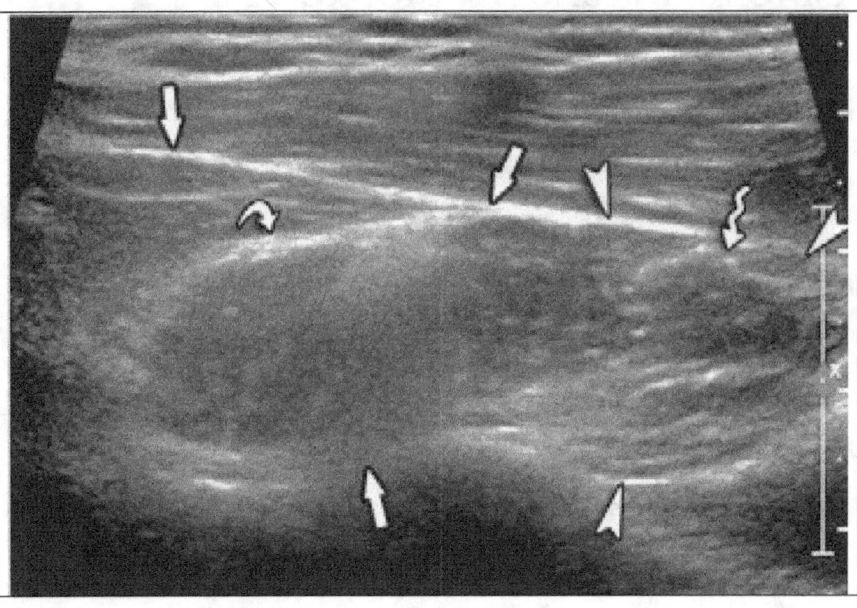

Figure-5.9D: Infraspinatus and teres minor (short axis). Corresponding ultrasound image shows infraspinatus (straight arrows) with central tendon (curved arrow) and teres minor (arrowheads) with more superficial tendon (squiggly arrow). Left side of image is cephalad

CHAPTER SIX
IMAGING DIAGNOSTIC MODALITES: COMPUTED TOMOGRAPHY

Computed tomography (CT-scan) is most often used following acute trauma as it allows for a comprehensive assessment of bone pathology.

A multi-detector CT-scan using sagittal and coronal reconstruction) can be used to assess the severity of humeral neck and head fractures. It can determine the number of fragments and their angle, the articular surface step-off and displacement. All of these factors can influence the prognosis and recovery time of a patient.

CT-scans are also used to assess a queried sterno-clavicular joint injury, as it clearly shows minute details of the fracture of dislocation.

The scapula is very complex. It consists of the body, the coracoid process, the acromion process and the gleno-humeral articular surface. A fracture in just the body can be treated conservatively, whilst fractures that affect the coracoid, acromion or articular surface can often necessitate surgery.

In cases of gleno-humeral dislocation, a CT-scan can reveal the location and size of the glenoid rim fragment which are important for planning a surgical intervention).

CT-scanning can be used to diagnose complex or hidden fractures of the gleno-humeral joint and scapula, as well as to assess dislocations and to monitor prosthetics.

CT-scans can reveal a number of important features including:

Complex fractures, and displacement.
Angulations and its severity.
Fracture lines and step-offs and fracture fragments in the joint itself.

CT-scan be useful in the assessment of tumors and dysplasia.

CT-scans can also be acquired in any possible plane allowing for simpler interpretation and surgical intervention.

CT arthrography is a suitable substitute for magnetic resonance arthrography. CT arthrography can be used to assess the labrum and rotator cuff.

The fact that 3D CT films can exclude the head of humerus means that the glenoid cavity aspect can be clearly visualized, and can aid surgical planning.

CT-scan is useful in assessing the integrity of the humerus and glenoid fossa, as well as the alignment and congruence of the whole joint.

CT arthrography can properly detail the articular surface, any loose bodies, and the whole labrum.

CHAPTER SEVEN
IMAGING DIAGNOSTIC MODALITES: MAGNETIC RESONANCE IMAGING (MRI)

MRI scanning is the most comprehensive method of visualizing the shoulder's soft tissues; the cartilage, labrum, muscles, tendons, ligaments and bursae.

MRI is useful for visualizing bone marrow, occult fractures, stress impact, contusion, edema, and bone erosion of the clavicle, degeneration of the AC joint, and the shape of the acromion, the presence of adhesive capsulitis, muscle wasting and changes associated with denervation.

MRI imaging is often used to obtain complex cross-sections of joints, and this makes it particularly useful in the shoulder joint.

MRI can reveal rotator cuff pathology and minute changes in the capsules and labrum including signs of gleno-humeral instability.

The application of IV or intra-articular gadolinium can help in visualizing lesions in the area, and bone injuries such as Hill-Sachs and Bankart lesions.

Standard protocols for shoulder imaging generally include:

T2-weighted sequencing with fat saturation in the oblique sagittal.
Oblique coronal and axial planes.
Obtaining information about gradient-echo and proton density in the axial plane.
T1-weighted sequences of the oblique sagittal and oblique coronal can allow assessment of fat atrophy of the cuff and bone marrow pathology.

The IV or intra-articular application of gadolinium can also be used to highlight fat saturation in T1-weighted architecture.

MRI IMAGING PLANES AND THEIR USES

The shoulder is imaged in three planes:

Coronal oblique images are obtained parallel to the supraspinatus tendon or perpendicular to the glenoid cavity if that tendon can not be visualized clearly because of retraction due to a full thickness tear.

Sagittal oblique images is perpendicular to supraspinatus tendon, and include medial aspect which enables evaluation of the rotator cuff muscle.

The axial or transverse images include the entire acromio-clavicular joint.

MRI sequences that can be used include:

Fat-suppressed T2-weighted with images obtained in the previously mentioned thee planes can help in recognizing tears. A fluid-filled cavity in the tendon is indicative of a cuff tear.

T1-weighted sagittal oblique can give information about wasting of the rotator cuff muscles, the degeneration of fat (a sign of adhesive capsulitis) and bone marrow health.

MR arthrography is generally regarded the gold standard for evaluating glenoid-labral tears and joint instability. It is the best method for visualizing 'superior labrum anterior-to-posterior' lesions, or SLAP lesions; these are an important subset of labral tears.

A fat-suppressed T1-weighted MRI and IV contrast is useful in the assessment of tumors and inflammatory arthropathies.

The 'short tau inversion recovery' (STIR) is the process that suppressed fat in the imaging, and is integral for imaging stress reactions and occult fractures.

For evaluation of the rotator cuff, imaging in the sagittal oblique and coronal oblique are necessary.

Transverse plane imaging enables viewing the biceps tendon (in the humeral groove), the subscapularis tendon and the glenoid-labrum.

Although T1-weighted sequences are best suited for imaging bony and fatty anatomy, T2-weighted sequences and proton-density scans are crucial for the assessment of the rotator cuff itself and the surrounding cartilage and neighboring bone marrow.

Assessment of the level of wasting in the rotator cuff muscles can provide information on rotator cuff tendinopathies. Surgery, and its proposed benefit, are closely linked to the degree of atrophy of the rotator cuff.

If the level of atrophy is very severe, surgery may not provide much improvement in quality of life.

The Goutallier et al (1994) and Fuchs et al (1999) (or modified Goutallier) classifications (Table-7.1) are used to assess the level of wasting present, through the use of CT and MRI scanning. However, there is a high degree of variability (both inter-observer and intra-observer), thereby making these classifications unreliable (Oh et al, 2010).

TABLE-7.1: THE GOUTALLIER ET AL (1994) AND FUCHS ET AL (1999) (OR MODIFIED GOUTALLIER) CLASSIFICATIONS OF MUSCLE STAGE
0 No fatty deposits Normal muscle
1 Some fatty streaks
2 Muscle >fat Moderately pathologic muscle
3 Muscle=fat Advanced degeneration
4 Muscle <fat

AC joint injury can be simply evaluated with a shoulder MRI scan. In the presence of an AC sprain, fluid or edema will be present in the joint space and in the surrounding soft tissue and bone marrow.

The visibility of the coracoid ligaments makes it easy to look for injury therein, as damage to these ligaments is often associated with AC dysfunction.

MRI is also useful in the assessment of post-traumatic distal clavicular osteolysis.

A stress reaction will be visible as contusion and edema in the marrow accompanied with stress fractures; this will be apparent well before traditional imaging could pick up signs of osteolysis.

INDICATIONS FOR AN MRI

Primary indications for MRI include diagnosis, exclusion, and grading of the following suspected conditions:

Rotator cuff pathology including complete, partial, recurrent, postoperative tears, and tendinitis, tear arthropathy.

Disorders of long head of biceps tendon including all types of tears, tendinopathy, tendinitis, subluxation, and dislocation.

Supraspinatus outlet disorders including acromion morphological issues, osacromiale, osteophytes, AC pathology, coraco-acromial ligament lesions, and subacromial bursitis.

Labral pathology including cysts, degeneration, all types of tears, SLAP lesions, Bankart lesions.

Rotator interval and biceps pulley pathologies.

Shoulder girdle muscle pathologies including hypertrophy, atrophy, denervation, and trauma, masses.

Cartilaginous pathologies including osteochondral fractures, osteochondritis dissecans, articular cartilage degeneration, fissures, and flaps.

Intra-articular bodies and synovial pathology including synovitis, bursitis, metaplasia, and neoplasia.

Marrow pathologies including osteonecrosis, marrow edema, and stress reactions.

Malignancy, masses, cysts, and infections of any tissue.

Congenital abnormalities including dysplasia, physiological variation.

Vascular pathology including entrapment, aneurysm, stenosis, and occlusion.

Neurological pathologies including entrapment, compression, masses, neuritis.

Magnetic resonance imaging of the shoulder may also be indicated in:

Arthritides including inflammation, infection, neuropathy, degeneration, crystallisation, post-trauma.
Frozen shoulder or adhesive capsulitis.
Tumors of bone and soft tissue (primary and secondary).
Fractures and dislocations.

Other indications of magnetic resonance imaging of the shoulder include:

Unresponsive shoulder pain and trauma to the shoulder
Impingement (Subacromial, subcoracoid, internal).
Gleno-humeral instability including chronic, recurrent, subacute, dislocation, and subluxation.
Shoulder dysfunction of overhead athletes.
Mechanical symptoms including catching, locking, snapping, crepitus.
Limited range of movement.
Edema, enlargement, masses or wasting.
Pre-arthroscopy and post-operative pain.

MRI FINDINGS IN SHOULDER IMPINGEMENT SYNDROME

The antero-lateral acromion is the most important factor in external compression of the cuff. Narrowing of the subacromial space can significantly increase the risk of impingement.

The MRI features of acromion morphology include:

The inferior acromion can be classified as follows: type I (flat); type II (gentle curving); type III (anterior hook); type IV (convexity).

Types II and III are particularly associated with impingement syndrome, with a scapula Y, X-ray can first show this.

The first or second image lateral to the AC joint (oblique sagittal plane) is used to determine acromion type (Figure-7.1A, B, and C, D).

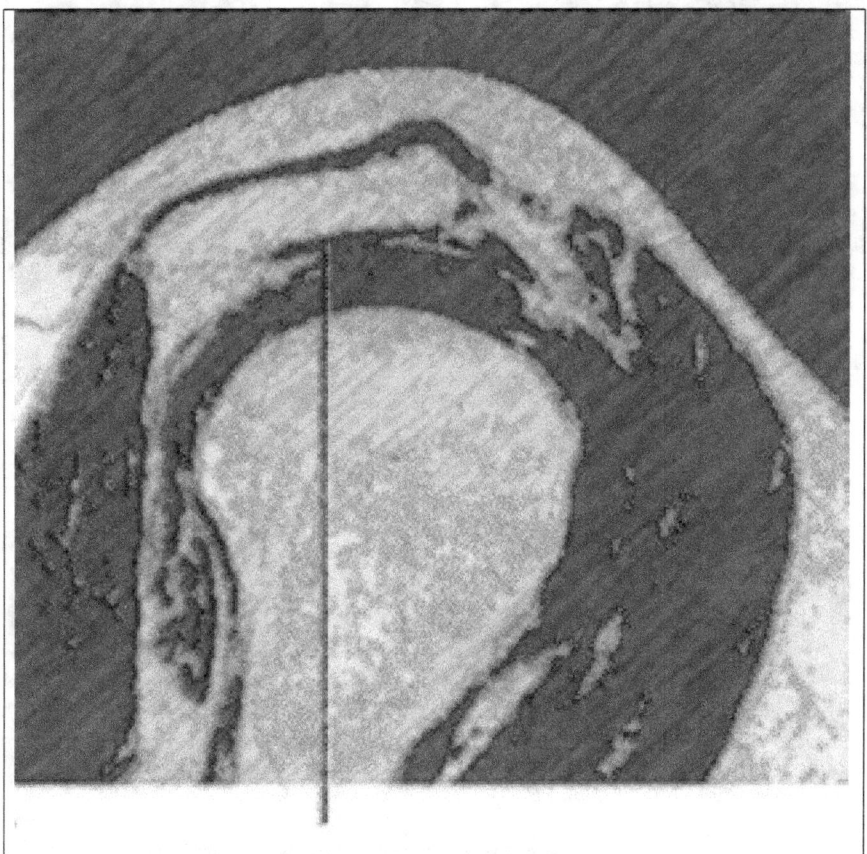

Figure-7.1A: Acromial typing using magnetic resonance imaging. Flat type I acromion.

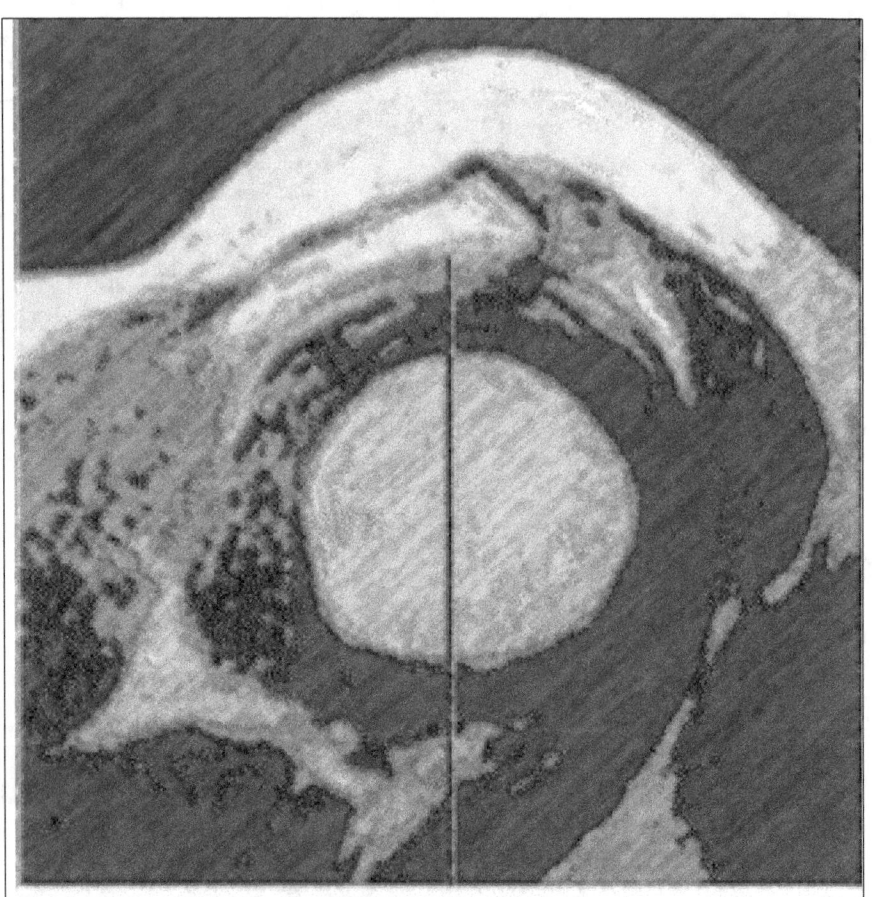

Figure-7.1B: Acromial typing using magnetic resonance imaging. Type II curved acromion

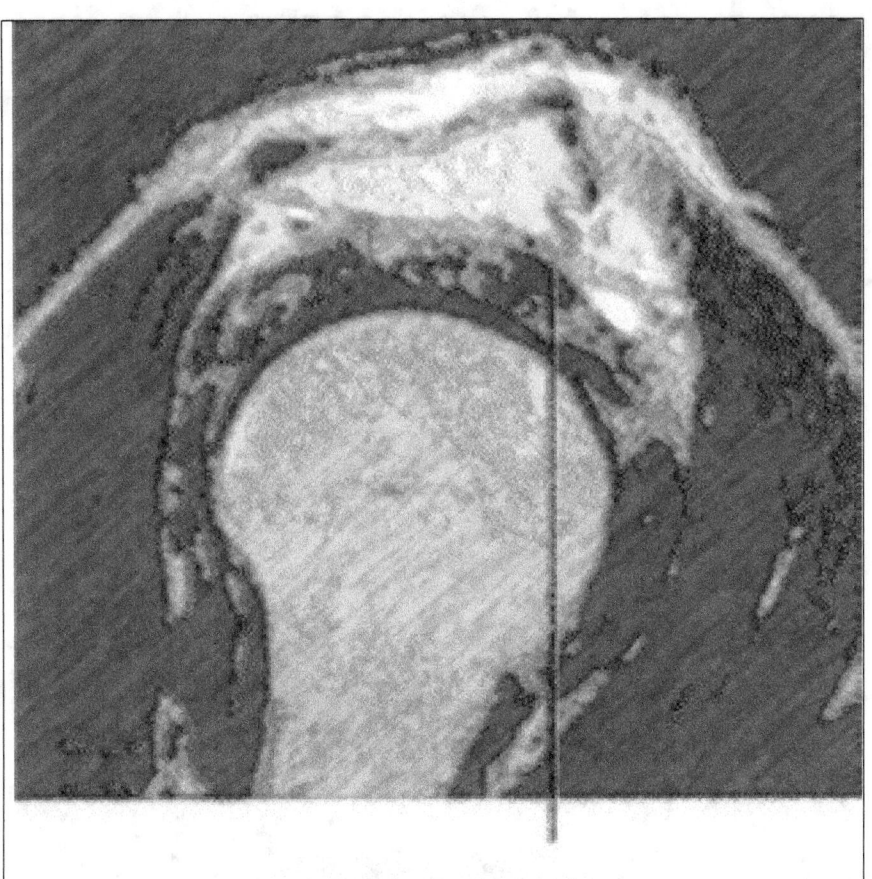

Figure-7.1C: Acromial typing using magnetic resonance imaging. Type III hooked acromion

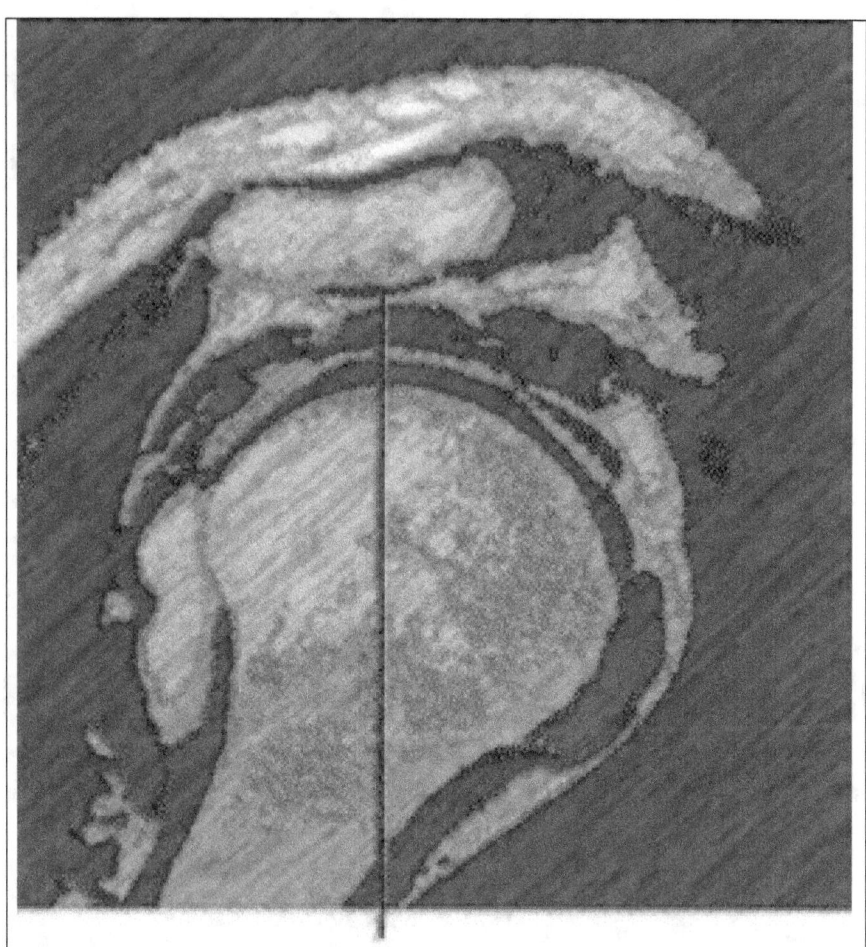

Figure-7.1D: Acromial typing using magnetic resonance imaging. Type IV convex acromion.

The acromial variations have even stronger association with impingement syndrome.

Anterior down-sloping of the scapula (Figure-7.2A) is associated with kyphosis, and can lead to narrowing and impingement. Figure-7.2B shows normal axis of acromion in the sagittal plane. Figure-7.2C shows lateral down-sloping of acromion with narrowing of osseous outlet. Figure-7.2D shows normal axis of acromion in coronal plane. Table-7.2 summarizes MRI evaluation of the osseous outlet and acromion.

Assessment for anterior down-sloping is performed using the sagittal plane. Anterior down-sloping describes the axis of the acromion in the sagittal plane and is independent of the undersurface of the acromion.

Osteophytes beneath the acromion. As the deltoid tendon slip attaches to the lateral acromion, this tendon slip can often be mistaken for a bone spur. However, a tendon slip will be dark on all pulse sequences, whereas an osteophyte will contain fatty marrow elements, and has fat signal intensity throughout (bright on T1). Figure-7.3A shows an acromial enthesiophyte. The Deltoid tendon slip can mimic an acromial enthesiophyte on MRI, but has no marrow and is dark throughout all sequences (Figure-7.3B).

An unfused osacromiale

The acromion is formed from a number of ossification centers, and fuses between the ages of 22 and 25. If an ossification centre does not fuse, the acromion can become unstable, with osteophytic lipping at the synchondrosis.

Unstable ossification centre acts as a fulcrum, displacing downwards when the deltoid contracts, thereby narrowing the subacromial space; this causes impingement. If this condition is not spotted and fixed during decompression surgery, it is liable to cause the decompression to fail.

Arthroscopic removal of fragments less than 4mm is generally recommended, as this does not affect the deltoid attachment or cause dysfunction. It is preferable to fuse larger fragments, as this likewise avoid weakness or dysfunction.

An unfused osacromiale can appear in different manners, depending on which centre does not fuse. Axial images best visualize an unfused osacromiale (Figure-7.4).

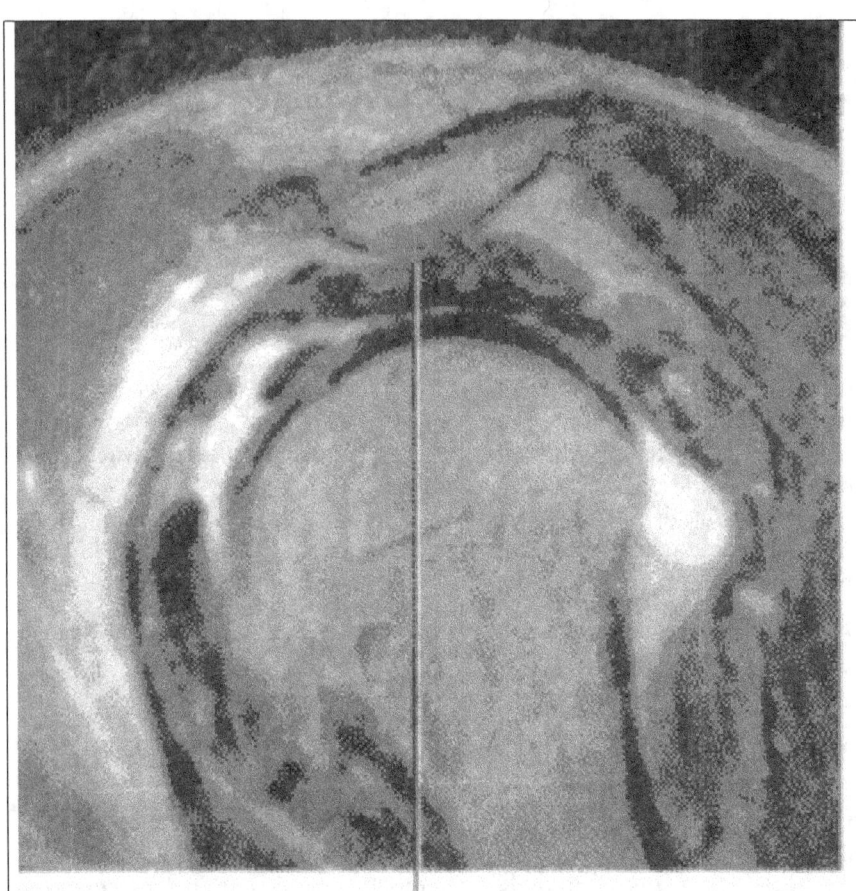

Figure-7.2A: Anterior down-sloping of the acromion narrowing the acromial-humeral distance, and causing rotator cuff impingement

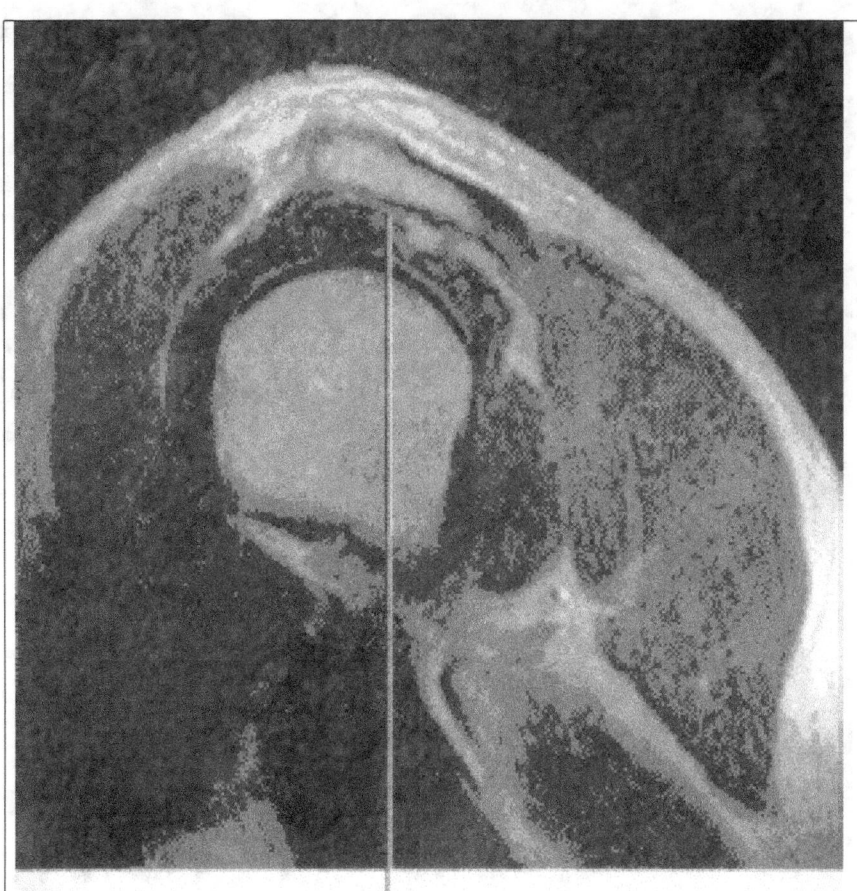

Figure-7.2B: Normal axis of acromion in the sagittal plane

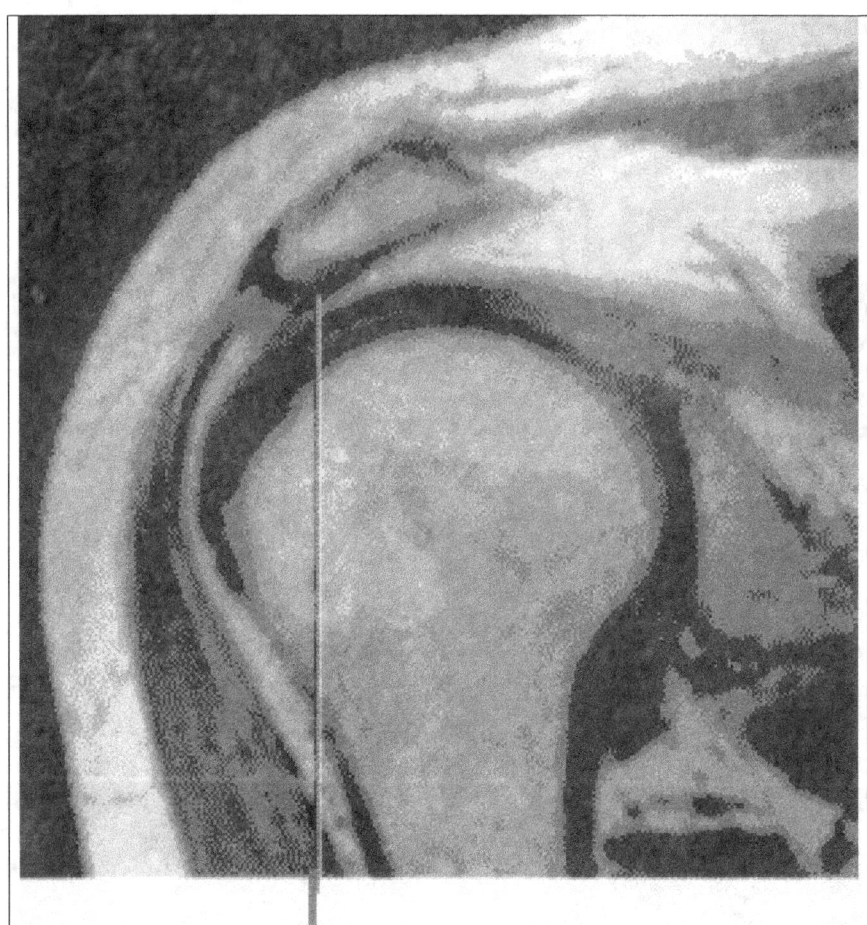

Figure-7.2C: Lateral down-sloping of acromion with narrowing of osseous outlet

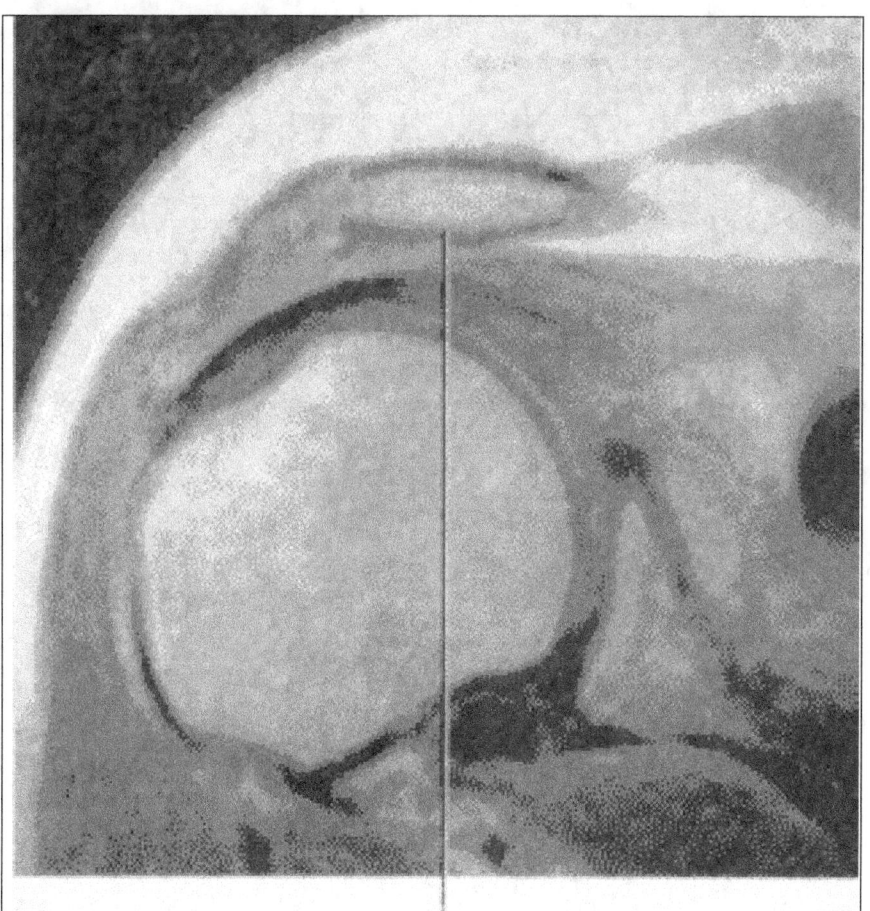

Figure-7.2D: Normal axis of acromion in coronal plane

TABLE-7.2: MRI EVALUATION OF THE OSSEOUS OUTLET AND ACROMION

Anatomic Part	Abnormality	Preferred MR Imaging Plane
Acromion	Type or configuration of undersurface (Types I, II, III, IV)	Sagittal: 1-2 images peripheral to AC joint
	Anterior down-sloping	Sagittal
	Lateral down-sloping	Coronal
	Enthesiophyte formation	Sagittal/coronal
	Osacromiale "double AC joint" sign	Axial: primary Sagittal/coronal-secondary
Acromio-clavicular (AC) joint	Osteoarthritis (mass effect on underlying cuff)	Coronal/sagittal
	AC joint separation (grades I, II, III)	Coronal
	Osteolysis of distal clavicle	Coronal
Coraco-acromial ligament	Thickening	Sagittal
	Calcification	Sagittal

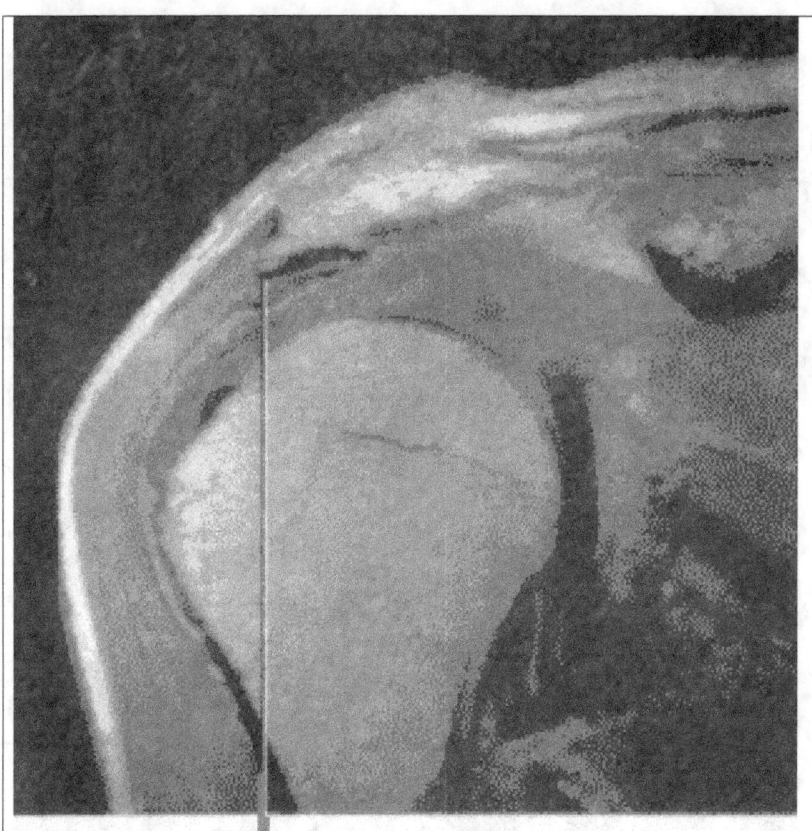

An enthesiophyte containing fatty marrow elements with a marrow signal intensity

Figure-7.3A: Acromial enthesiophyte. Coronal T1-weighted image demonstrates an enthesiophyte extending from the undersurface of the acromion, causing impingement. An enthesiophyte contains fatty marrow elements and has a marrow signal intensity on MRI

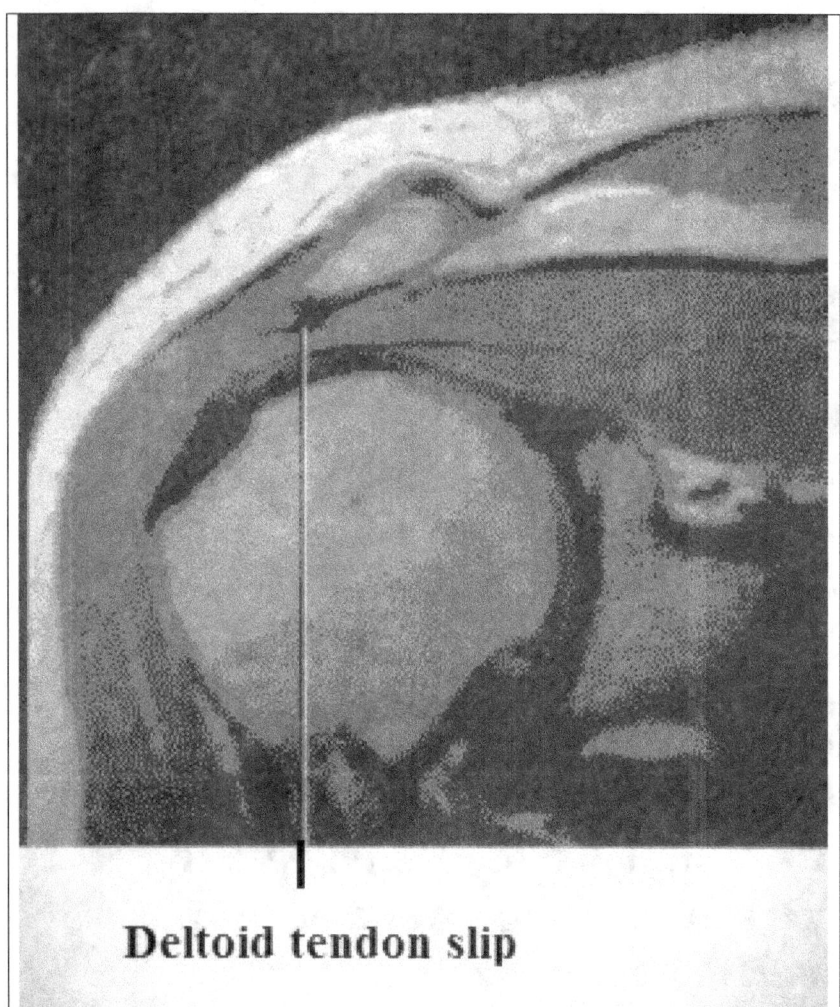

Figure-7.3B: The Deltoid tendon slip can mimic an acromial enthesiophyte on MRI, but has no marrow and is dark throughout all sequences

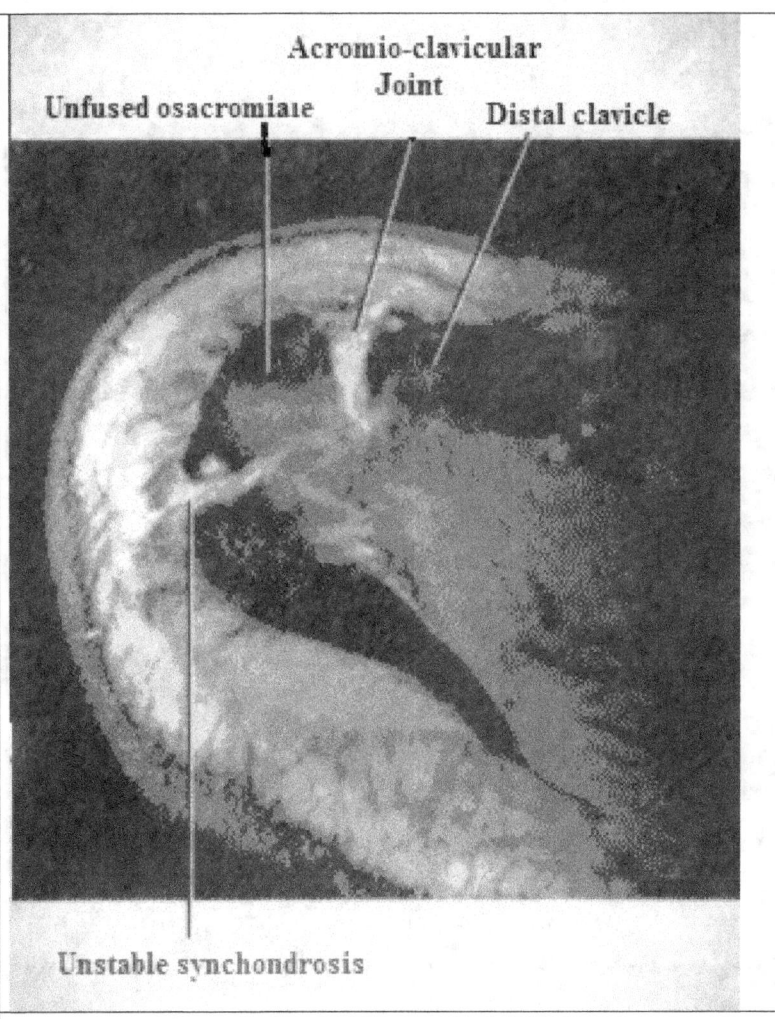

Figure-7.4A: Osacromiale on MR imaging. Unfused osacromiale on axial MRI images. The presence of a fluid signal within the synchondrosis and subcortical cysts suggests that the unfused ossification center is unstable, acting as a "hinge", resulting in shoulder impingement

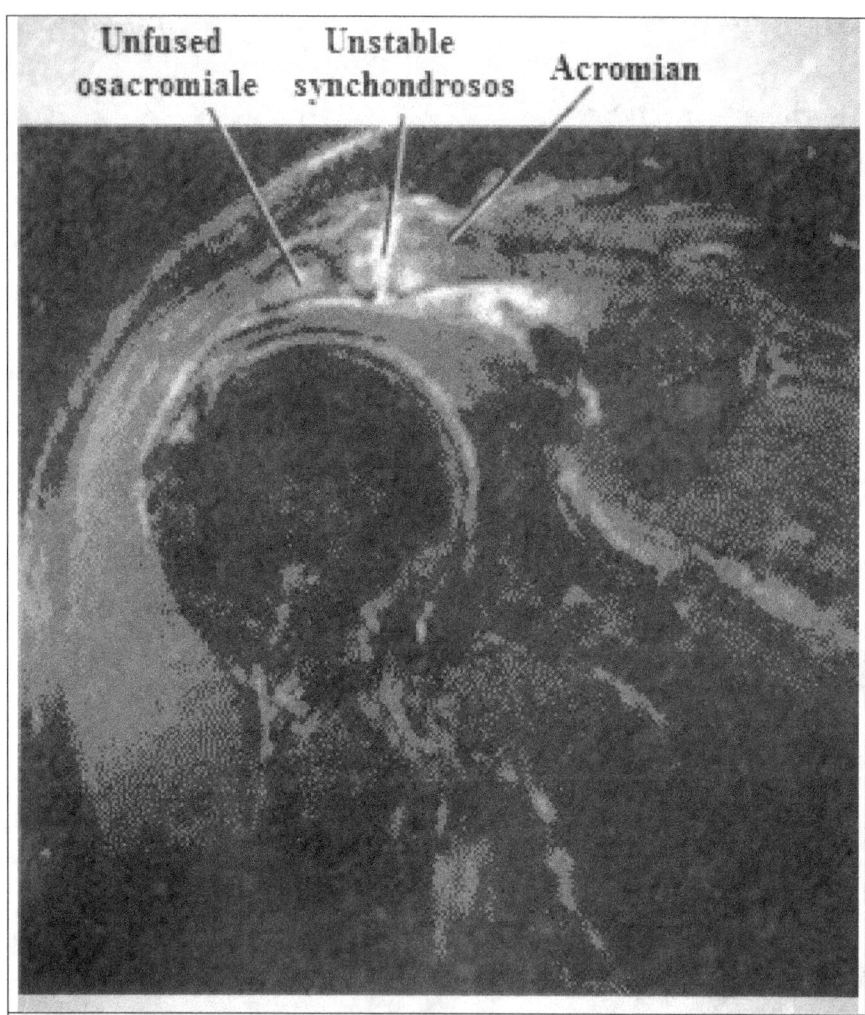

Figure-7.4B: Osacromiale on MR imaging. Unfused osacromiale on coronal MRI images. The presence of a fluid signal within the synchondrosis and subcortical cysts suggests that the unfused ossification center is unstable, acting as a "hinge", resulting in shoulder impingement

The appearance of an unfused osacromiale on sagittal or coronal planes can appear much like an AC joint, and can be interpreted as such. If both AC joint and unfused osacromiale are on the same film, this appears as "The double AC joint sign" (Figure-7.5). This is most often the case two or three slices posterior to the real AC joint. If there is fluid in the synchondrosis or edema around it, this is indicative of pseudoarthrosis or a fibrous union; this points to an unstable joint.

An unfused osacromiale can often appear like a fracture of the acromion. However, in an osacromiale, the accessory ossicle usually appears triangular with sclerotic margins, forming a synchondrosis that is always perpendicular to the long axis of the acromion. Conversely, in a fracture, the angle is usually oblique, and the margins tend to be irregular and non sclerotic.

Imaging of the shoulder will often reveal pathology of the Acromio-clavicular joint. In patients over 40, arthritis is a common finding, whilst younger patients may have joint separation or osteolysis following acute trauma. These pathologies can appear similar, but a combination of history and imaging can usually distinguish them (Table-7.3).

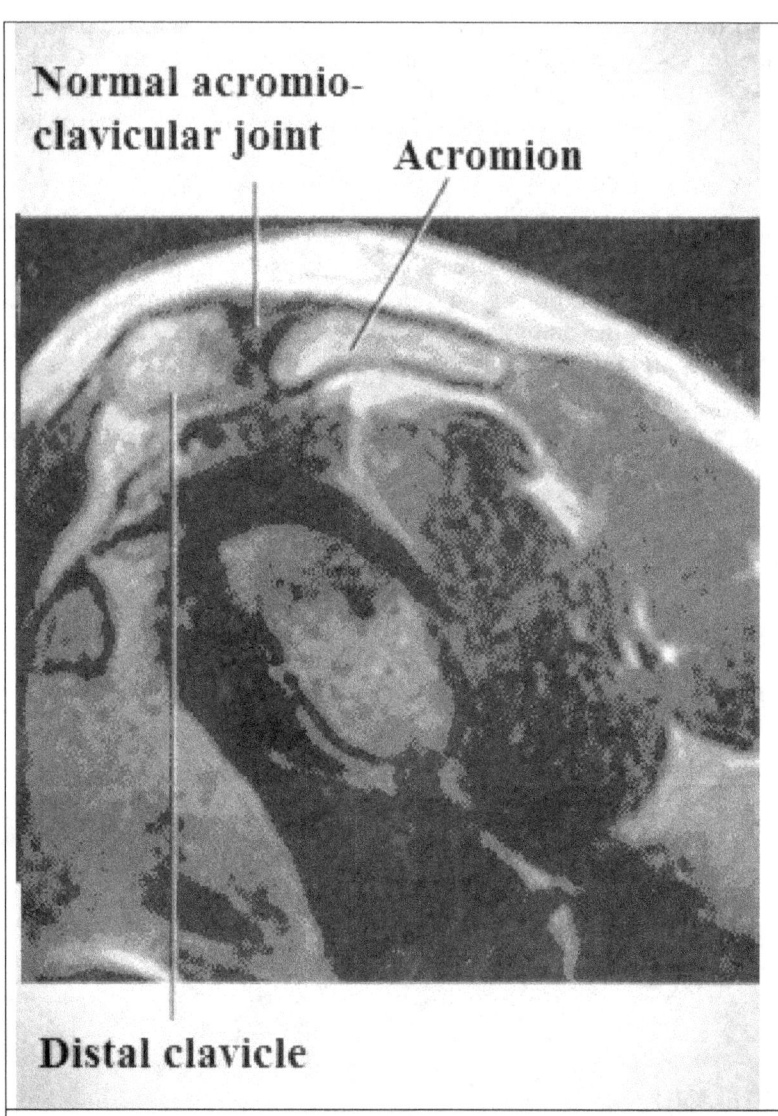

Figure-7.5A: Double acromio-clavicular joint. Oblique sagittal images at the level of the normal acromio-clavicular joint

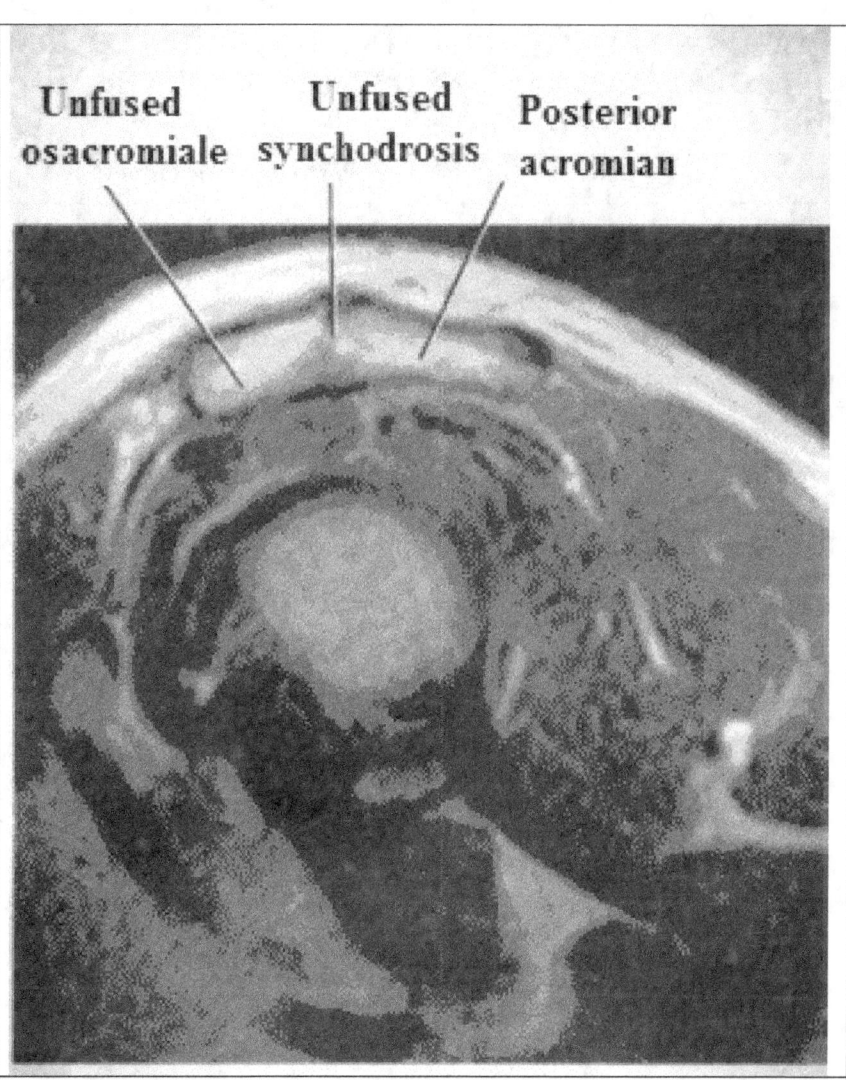

Figure-7.5B: The unfused osacromiale appears as a second acromio-clavicular joint on a more peripheral image easily mistaken for the true acromio-clavicular joint

TABLE-7.3: ACROMIO-CLAVICULAR JOINT OSTEOARTHRITIS VERSUS OSTEOLYSIS OF THE DISTAL CLAVICLE

	Osteoarthritis	Post-traumatic Osteolysis
Patient	Typically > 40	Young athlete
Symptoms	Minimally symptomatic or asymptomatic	Painful
Etiology	No history of trauma	Acute trauma: Repetitive micro-trauma (weight-lifters)
Location of involvement	Both sides of joint	Isolated to distal clavicle
Radiographic Findings	Joint space narrowing Osteophyte formation Subchondral cyst/sclerosis	Acute Soft tissue swelling Demineralization distal clavicle Loss cortical margin distal clavicle AC joint appears widened Chronic Reconstitution distal clavicle Subchondral sclerosis/cysts
MR findings	Joint space narrowing Osteophyte formation Subchondral cyst/sclerosis Capsular hypertrophy Joint effusion	Marrow edema distal clavicle Capsular hypertrophy Adjacent soft tissue edema Loss of dark cortical line AC joint widening

Osteoarthritis of the acromio-clavicular usually affects both sides of the acromio-clavicular. MRI imaging findings include capsular hypertrophy, effusion and edema of the surrounding soft tissue. Other frequent findings include osteophytes, subchondral marrow changes and subchondral cysts.

Other causes of edema are acromio-clavicular separation and inflammatory arthritis.

Arthritis of the acromio-clavicular can cause extrinsic impingement on the rotator cuff, but the acromio-clavicular joint is not as implicated as the acromion in causing impingement.

Degeneration of the acromio-clavicular joint and the associated effects on the rotator cuff can be seen most clearly using MRI (Figure-7.6).

Joint effusion and peri-capsular edema are often linked to acromio-clavicular synovitis and symptomatic osteoarthritis.

Osteoarthritis of the acromio-clavicular joint is best detected on coronal projections. On this coronal T1-weighted image there is capsular hypertrophy, loss of the normal cortex of the clavicle and neighboring acromion and an inferiorly facing osteophyte resulting in a mass effect on the underlying rotator cuff.

Post-traumatic osteolysis of the distal portion of the clavicle tends to develop after mild or moderate injury to the acromio-clavicular joint. This painful pathology is often observed in patients who have repeated micro-trauma, such as weightlifters.

It is different to osteoarthritis in that it occurs in the young and the fit, following trauma, and causes acute (potentially severe) pain; osteoarthritis occurs in the old, has no history of trauma, and causes mild progressive pain.

The radiographs of initial post-traumatic osteolysis show soft tissue swelling around the AC, demineralization and a reduced cortical margin of the distal clavicle (Figure-7.7A).

Immediately following injury, the AC joint will widen, but with time the clavicle reconstructs. Subchondral sclerosis and subchondral cysts may be a chronic that lingers after recovery.

In initial osteolysis, MRI images may marrow edema in the distal 1-3cm of the clavicle, and a lost cortical margin. Joint effusion, capsular hypertrophy and peri-capsular edema are common signs.

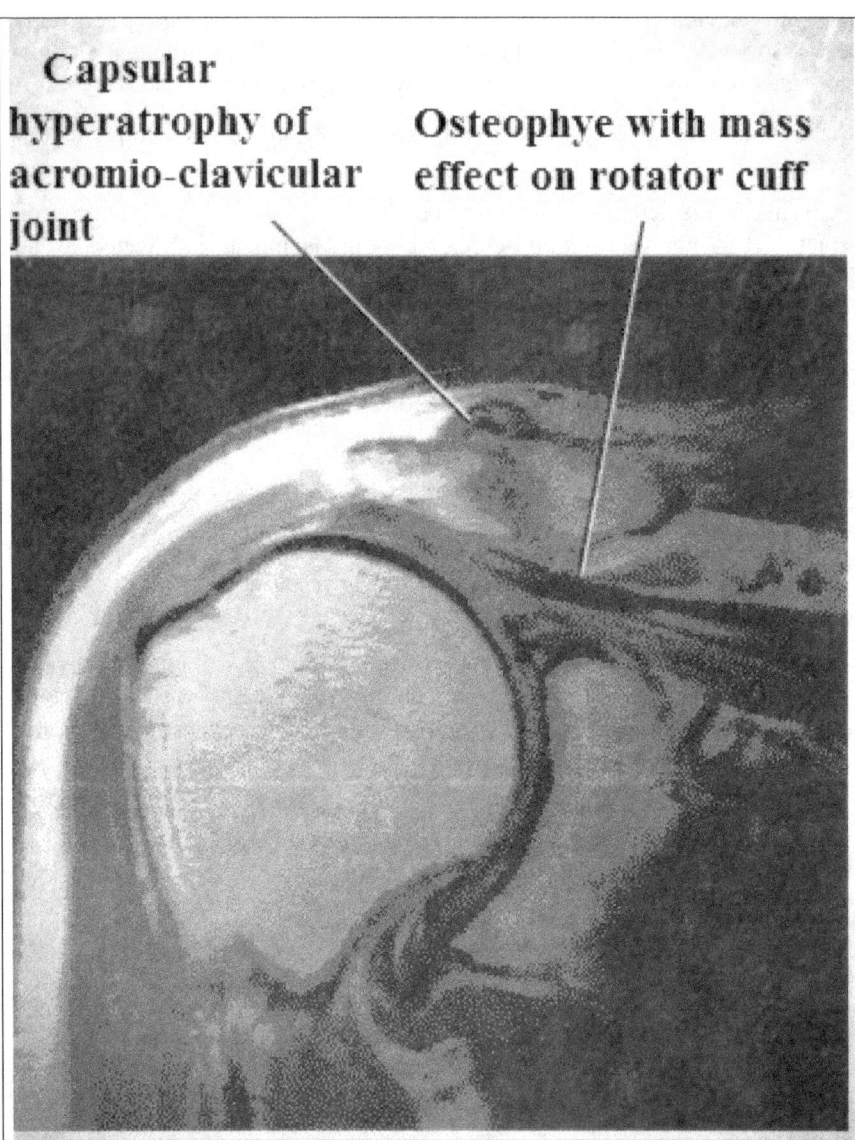

Figure-7.6: Osteoarthritis of the acromio-clavicular joint

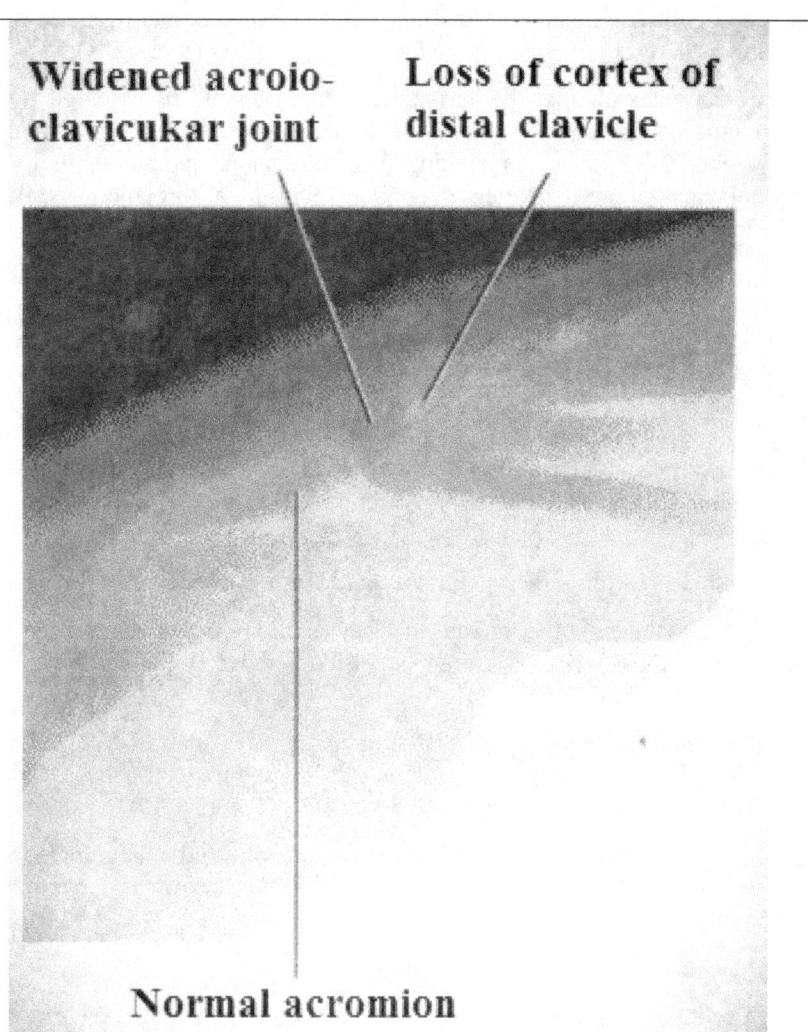

Figure-7.7A: Osteolysis of the distal clavicle. Radiograph of the acromio-clavicular joint showing soft tissue swelling superiorly. There is widening of the acromio-clavicular joint, loss of the normal cortical white line of the clavicle and subchondral cysts

Later in the disease, the acromio-clavicular joint might widen, the capsular hypertrophy will reduce but remain and the cortex will become irregular or subchondral sclerosis of the distal clavicle will develop ((Figure-7.7B).

Following shoulder trauma, the acromio-clavicular should be assessed for joint separation or fractures. A fracture will appear as a dark line on an MRI (both T1 and T2) with accompanying marrow edema. Separation of the acromio-clavicular can be categorized according to a three-point scale (Figure-7.8).

The coracoid ligament is an integral part of the osseous outlet, lying over the anterior portion of the supraspinatus tendon and the rotator interval. It runs from the coracoid process (anterior) to the acromion (posterior).

Oblique sagittal MRI images are the best means of identifying it, and it is between 2 and 3mm thick (Figure-7.9A).

If the ligament becomes hypertrophied, thickened or calcified it can result in extrinsic impingement on the anterior rotator cuff (Figure-7.9B).

Coraco-humeral Impingement (Subcoracoid Impingement)

Subcoracoid impingement is an unusual cause of impingement, and is a result of subscapularis tendon entrapped inside a reduced coraco-humeral space.

A healthy coraco-humeral space is 11mm in diameter (in an axial MRI); if it becomes less than 7mm, the subscapularis can become trapped between the head of humerus and the coracoid resulting in a tear (Figure-7.10).

Surgical management involves both repair of the tendon and enlargement of the coraco-humeral space. If the subscapularis tendon is torn in isolation, suspicion of a coraco-humeral impingement should be raised.

MRI appearance of the normal Rotator Cuff

Assessment of supraspinatus muscle is best performed in the oblique coronal and sagittal planes (Figure-7.11A, B). Axial images are also helpful. In a healthy adult, the muscle should fill the supraspinatus fossa, and has an intermediate T1 and T2 signal. The muscle mass should match teres minor and infraspinatus. The healthy musculo-tendinous junction is located at the 12 o'clock position of the head of humerus.

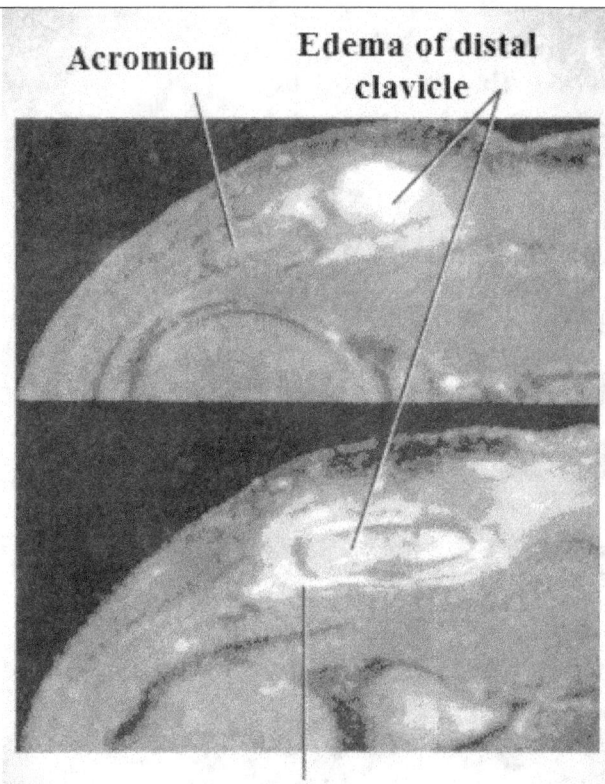

Figure-7.7B: Osteolysis of the distal clavicle. The changes are more marked on the clavicular side of the joint. Sequential coronal T2-weighted images through the acromio-clavicular joint showed marrow edema isolated to the distal clavicle with surrounding soft tissue edema, mild periostitis, and a small joint effusion. The signal intensity within the adjacent acromion is normal

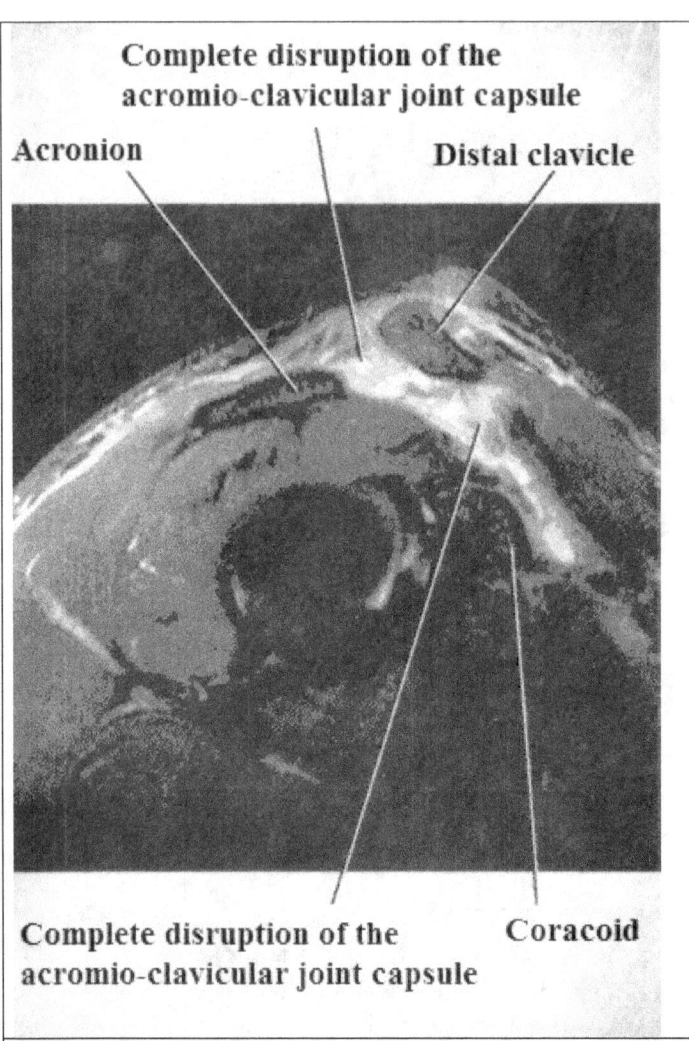

Figure-7.8 Grade III acromio-clavicular joint separation. There is complete disruption of the acromio-clavicular joint capsule and the coraco-clavicular ligaments. There is also elevation of the distal clavicle

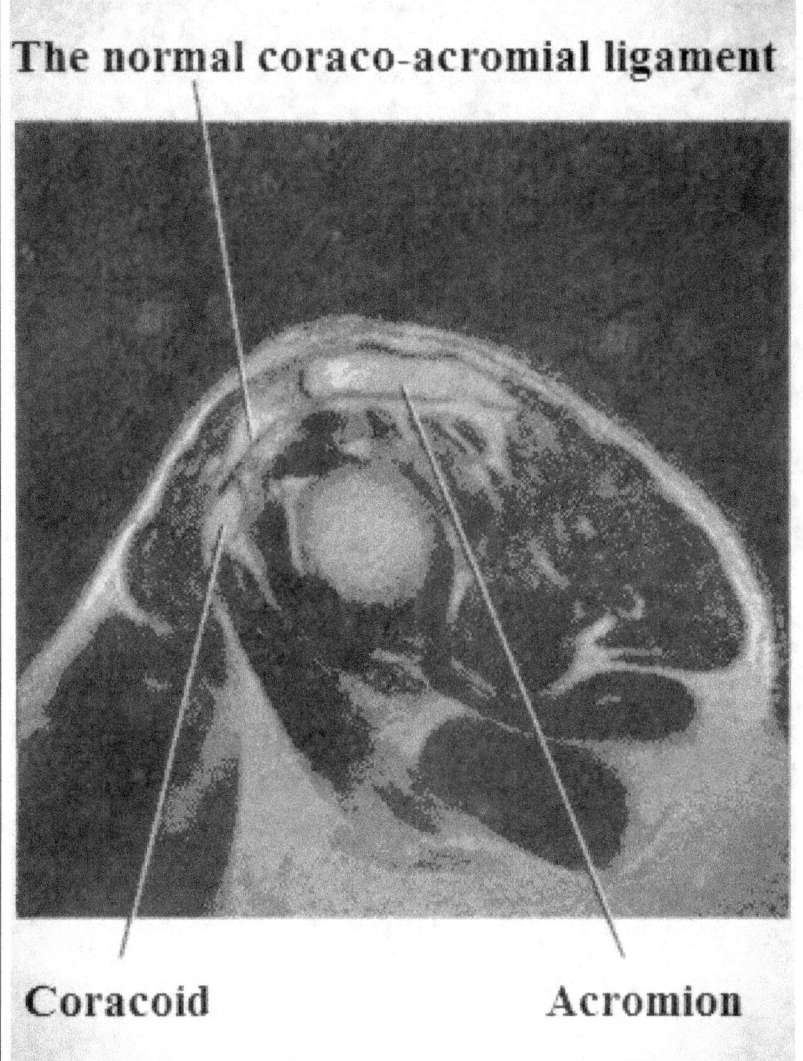

Figure-7.9A: The normal coraco-acromial ligament is smooth and less than 3 mm thick and is best seen on oblique sagittal projections. It extends from the coracoid process to the acromion

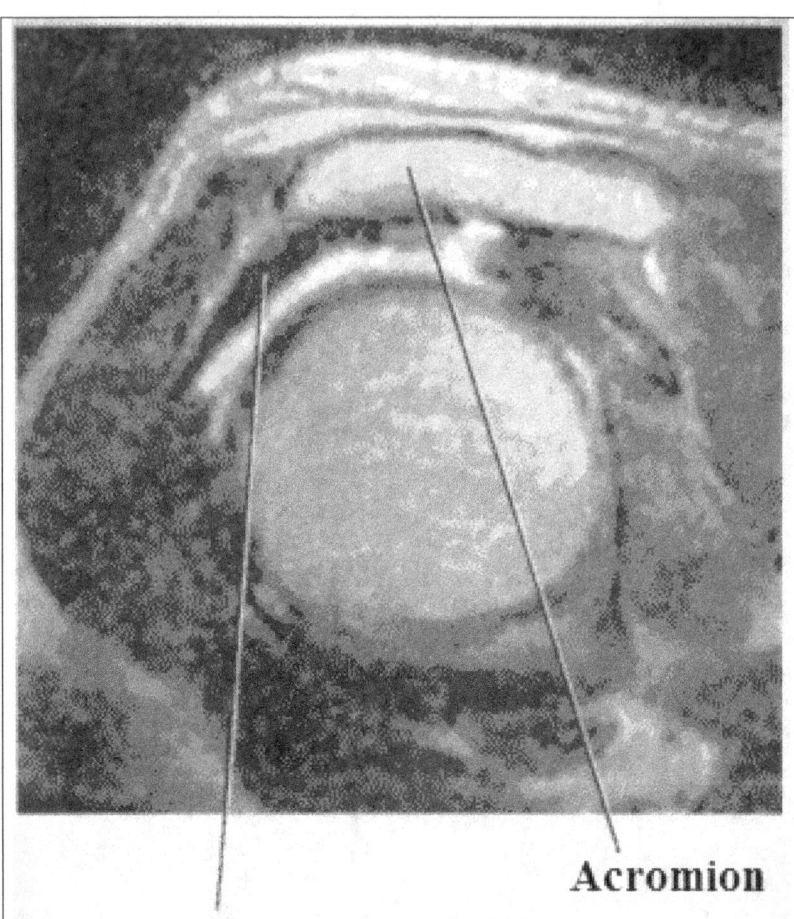

Figure-7.9B: Marked thickening of the coraco-acromial ligament near its acromial attachment. Thickening or nodularity of the ligament can result in impingement of the rotator cuff.

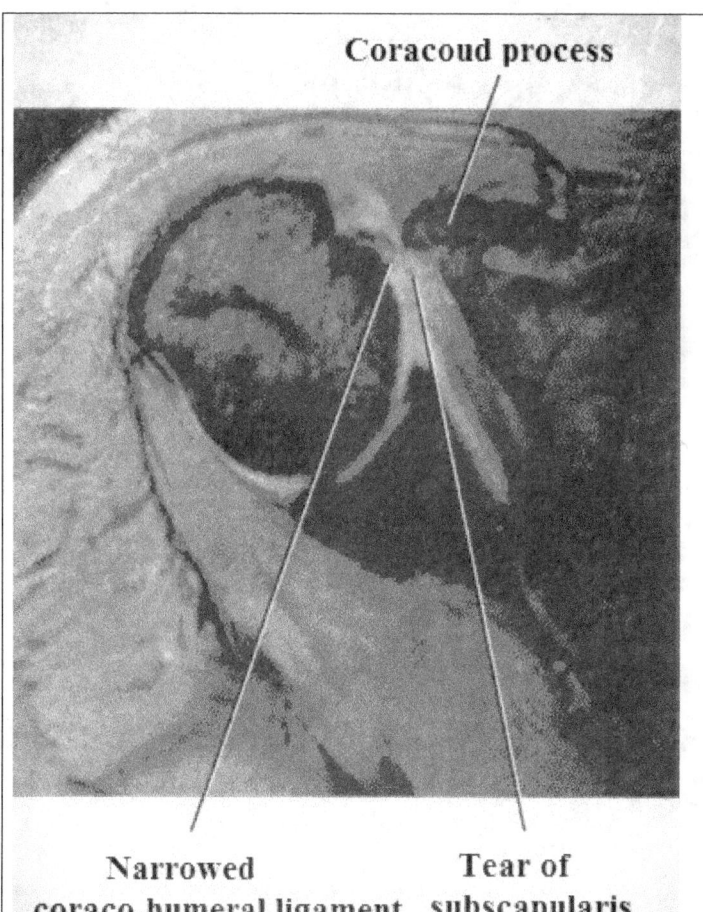

Figure-7.10: Coraco-humeral impingement. Axial T2-weighted MRI showing a narrowed coraco-humeral distance, causing entrapment of the subscapularis tendon and partial tearing of the tendon near its attachment to the lesser tuberosity

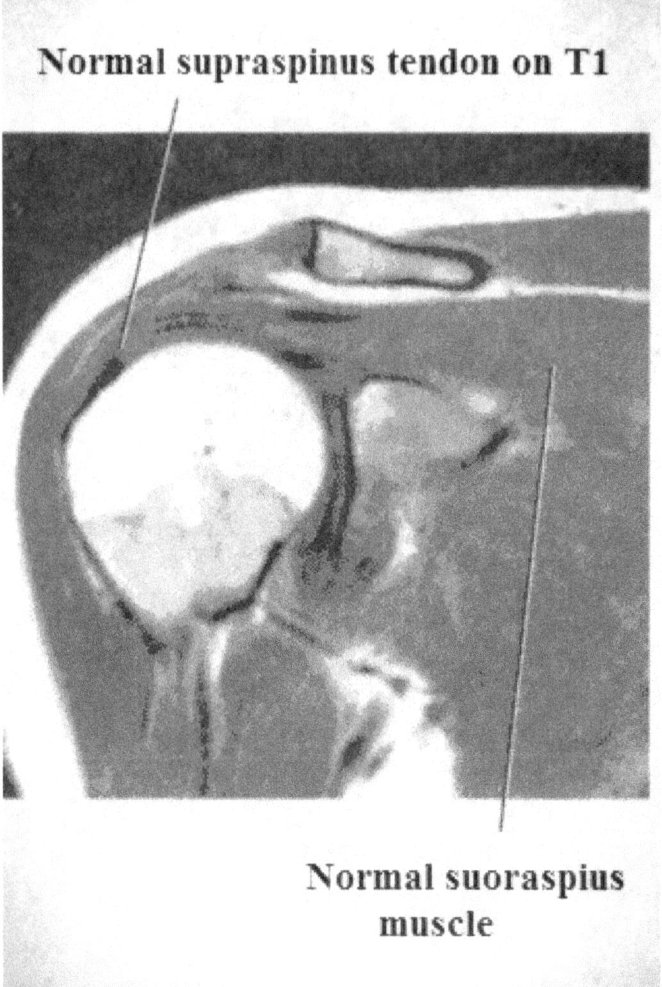

Figure-7.11A: The normal supraspinatus tendon shows low T1 and T2 signal, oriented in the horizontal plane. The normal musculo-tendinous junction is in the 12 o'clock position of the humeral head. Muscle is intermediate signal intensity on both T1 and T2-weighted images

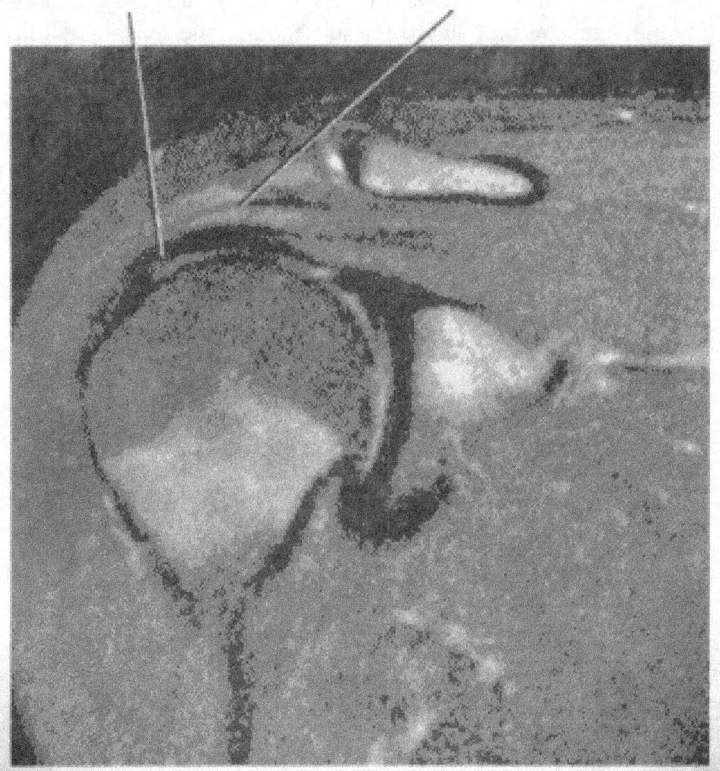

Figure-7.11B: The normal supraspinatus tendon shows low T1 and T2 signal, oriented in the horizontal plane. The normal musculo-tendinous junction is in the 12 o'clock position of the humeral head. Muscle is intermediate signal intensity on both T1 and T2-weighted images

Like the supraspinatus, the teres minor and infraspinatus muscle are best assessed using the oblique coronal and oblique sagittal planes. In the films, the muscles fill the infraspinatus fossa, and appear to taper peripherally and have a similar musculo-tendinous junction as supraspinatus. In coronal plane images, infraspinatus and supraspinatus can be distinguished by orientation; supraspinatus is horizontal, infraspinatus is oblique.

The sensitivity and specificity of MRI in its ability to detect rotator cuff tears varies from 88% to 100%. T2-weighted coronal or sagittal images are best suited for imaging supraspinatus and infraspinatus pathology, whereas axial T2-weighted images are best suited for subscapularis lesions. The following table categorizes rotator cuff disease (Table-7.4).

TABLE-7.4: MRI APPEARANCE OF ROTATOR CUFF PATHOLOGY	
Cuff Pathology	**Appearance on MRI**
Normal tendon	Dark on T1 and T2
Tendonopathy	Thickening of tendon
	Intermediate signal T1/T2
Calcific tendinitis	Globular decreased signal T1/T2 within tendon; often with surrounding soft tissue edema
	Thickened tendon; intermediate signal T1/T2
	"Blooming" artifact on gradient echo
Partial-thickness tear	Fluid signal/gadolinium extending partially through tendon superior to inferior
	Bursal/articular/interstitial
	Associated intramuscular cyst
	No retraction of tendon
Full-thickness tear	Fluid extending completely through tendon top to bottom
	Retraction of tendon
	Gap/discontinuity in tendon
Musculo-tendinous retraction	Measured as the length of the medial-to-lateral tendon gap
Fatty atrophy	Grade: mild/moderate/severe
	Streaks of high signal on T1—irreversible
	Loss of muscle bulk relative to other rotator cuff muscles on sagittal imaging (reversible)

Limitations of MRI

Contraindications to performing an MRI include:

Pacemakers to defibrillators.
Aneurysm clips.
Metallic bodies.
Cochlear implants or other electronic implants.

A plain radiograph should be obtained if there is any suspicion of a metallic object being present.

Orthopedic surgical materials become MRI-suitable in a matter of six weeks; after this point, as long as there is enough tissue to support the material, an MRI can be performed.

As with other medical procedures, it is important to weigh up the risks and benefits of an MRI to make sure that the correct course of action is taken.

MRI imaging is also cautioned in the case of claustrophobia. In such cases, IV sedation (preserving consciousness) should be given to those below the age of six or who demonstrate uncontrollable symptoms. As with all sedation, it is important to monitor vital signs throughout. Open MRI systems have been proposed as an alternative for those suffering from claustrophobia, but the resolution of these systems lag behind those of traditional MRI machines.

CHAPTER EIGHT: TREATMENT OF SHOULDER IMPINGEMENT

NON-OPERATIVE TREATMENT

Non-operative therapies interventions for shoulder impingement include:

Rest, cold, heat, acupuncture, trans-cutaneous nerve stimulation, stretching and exercise.

Education can help in recovery. A patient generally needs a good understanding of the disease, how it developed, and what they should expect from treatment.

Oral NSAIDS: In primary care, a suitable first approach is one of rest and analgesia. Oral NSAIDS have been shown to be effective. However, awareess of the possible side effects and contraindications of NSAIDS is mandatory.

NSAIDs may also be injected into the subacromial space, significantly improving symptoms with minimal side effects (as can accompany corticosteroid injections) (157).

Corticosteroid injections to the affected joint may provide significant relief to shoulder pain. Pain is especially reduced (in the acute and subacute phases) when injections were used in combination with exercise.

Ultrasound guided injections are also useful in improving analgesia and recovery.

Current recommendations suggest that corticosteroid injections should be used in subacute or acute tendinitis; the benefit in such situations is clearer cut than in a chronic presentation.

Exercise treatment has been reported in several studies to be very effective in improving recovery in impingement patients.

Strengthening exercises for rotator cuff and scapular muscles are generally combined with stretching exercises for the shoulder soft tissues. These treatments can help both pain and functionality of the affected joint.

The choice of therapy depends largely on the specialty of the treating physician. There are no clearly-defined rules on what exercises are best, and there is no consensus on how to best target muscle groups.

Non operative interventions are a practicable alternative or supportive treatment for most patients.

If patients fail to improve with non operative therapy, surgical intervention is recommended. However, early surgery does not improve prognosis.

Surgical interventions are generally aim at adjusting the anatomical abnormality by enlarging the subacromial space and eliminating impingement of the cuff. The anterior curve of the acromion is remodeled, artificially creating a type I-like acromion. This acromioplasty is combined with the removal of osteophytes from the AC and resection of the coraco-acromial ligament and subacromial bursa.

Postoperative rehabilitation aims at improving function and preventing re-emergence of the problem. The available evidence supports the use of exercise treatment in the management of subacromial impingement.

Exercise reduces pain, and also improves shoulder function. Further research still needs to be done on individual regimens and how they perform in isolation, and what exactly makes an effective exercise therapy.

Laser is a monochromatic and non-ionizing beam that can impact cellular function. It can be used to stimulate tissues and to reduce inflammation and pain. It is not currently advised due to the lack of concrete evidence of significant benefit.

Ultrasound can be used to create a deep thermal or non-thermal effect in tissues to which it is applied. It has been posited that the EM fields generated can increase oxygen dispersal, cause vasodilatation and alleviate pain. However, there is little evidence supporting its use in shoulder impingement, and it is no more effective than a placebo.

Massage is another non-invasive method of analgesia in shoulder pain. By handling myofascial trigger points in muscles or soft tissue, masseuses can improve patient's symptoms and function better than in those who receive no treatment (180).

Acupuncture has been suggested to improve blood or energy flow in the body, possibly overriding nerve signals or releasing homogenous analgesics. It has been suggested as an alternative treatment for longstanding shoulder pain.

Platelet-rich plasma injections involve injecting autologous blood fractions (highly concentrated in platelets) into the subacromial space. This has been posited to improve regeneration of the joint, through the action of growth factors made by platelets. There is little to no evidence for the use of these injections in shoulder pathology, and its use is not recommended.

Surgery is used for patients who have not improved with non-surgical methods.

Neer has revolutionized the surgical field when he who used decompression of the cuff and acromion.

Previous procedures such as extensive resection or acromionectomy were abandoned in favor of Neer's approach which involves remodeling of the acromion to relieve pressure on the rotator cuff. This procedure enlarges the subacromial space and thereby alleviates impingement.

Acromioplasty aims at recreating a type I acromion through reshaping the curve and removing osteophytes; the coraco-acromial ligament or subacromial bursa may also be resected.

Conventional open acromioplasty is performed through a 9cm incision made from the anterior acromion to the lateral coracoid process. An osteotome is used to remove the inferior aspect of the acromion, including the whole attachment for the coraco-acromial ligament. Bony prominences are also excised, as is the distal clavicle if there is concomitant arthritis.

Arthroscopic acromioplasty was first used by Ellman in 1985, first called "arthroscopic subacromial decompression". Ellman used a series of portals (antero-lateral, postero-lateral and posterior) to access the bursa and debride it, thereby releasing the coraco-acromial ligament.

A powered burr is used in the procedure. This arthroscopic method allows the surgeon to better seen the inferior aspect of the arch, and any accompanying abrasion or causes of impingement. As this operation replicates the results of open acromioplasty, the choice of procedure is often left to the surgeon to decide, and often to the patient's preference.

Bursectomy, or arthroscopic debridement, has been shown to give similar effects whether performed in isolation or alongside acromioplasty. Some studies have found that debridement alone is sufficient in many cases, especially for those with partial cuff tears; up to 79% experience good to excellent long-term outcomes with debridement alone.

CHAPTER NINE
THE ROLE OF SHOULDER IMAGING IN DIAGNOSIS, STAGING AND MANAGEMENT OF SHOULDER IMPINGEMENT

The diagnosis of shoulder impingement is primarily clinical. Early diagnosing and treatment of impingement helps in avoiding the risk of impingement worsening with time or progressing to tears or ruptures.

Improvements in imaging provided better assessment and understanding of shoulder pathologies.

There are many treatment options available, and physicians need to talk to the patient in order to establish a treatment plan that works best for them.

Plain radiographs are a vital first-line test, but are liable to appear normal in the early stages of the disease. Other modalities, MRI imaging, ultrasound scan are excellent at early diagnosis, and can supplement X-rays if necessary.

Radiographs can suggest impingement especially in the presences of structures that invade the supraspinatus outlet such as osteophytes, and tilted acromion.

Radiography can also detect the presence of a type III acromion, or a hooked acromion, which can increase one's risk of developing impingement and developing a cuff tear; it is clearly visible in a modified Y projection film.

However, X-ray films can often be normal in acute cuff tears, and radiography's ability to detect tears early is limited especially in stage I, where edema and inflammation are the core signs.

Although radiography can aid in planning therapy, one study found that radiography had no impact on health outcomes for impingement patients, suggesting that it alone is not sufficient.

Once the disease has progressed, the superiorly-located humerus and humeral head (acromio-humeral distance >7mm), it can be detected on AP radiographs.

Chronic cuff tears can cause remodeling of the bony architecture especially of the greater tuberosity which can be associated with pitting, notching, acromial concavity and reactive osteophytosis in the gleno-humeral joint. This may be detected on a radiograph.

Although useful in trauma and other conditions, the inability to detect edema and occult fractures ultimately limit radiography in the diagnosis of rotator cuff pathology.

Ultrasonography is inexpensive, noninvasive, readily available and incredibly effective imaging modality; some have suggested it is the most important imaging tool for shoulder pathologies, and should be used first line with radiography (218).

Ultrasonography is a very effective way of diagnosing and monitoring shoulder impingement, and recent technological advances have improved its efficacy.

Ultrasonography is already extensively used in the assessment of structures of the shoulder, along with accompanying pathologies of the rotator cuff and the surrounding tissue.

The accuracy of ultrasonography is between 91% (for partial tears) and 100% (for full tears), being as accurate as MRI. Ultrasonography is also able to assess the shoulder whilst in movement; this dynamic evaluation is an invaluable tool for diagnosis.

Dynamic ultrasonography can be performed to assess the joint in movement, ability unique to the imaging modality, and it can diagnose conditions that no other method can diagnose.

The dynamic exam can reveal what is being impinged and whether the humeral head migrates upwards; these are useful clues for the potential cause of impingement. Even static ultrasound is useful in detecting narrowing, bursitis, tendinopathy, effusion and synovitis. This can be complemented with Doppler ultrasonography to assess vascular function if active synovitis is present.

As a staging procedure, ultrasonography is able to pick up tendinosis and bursitis, determining whether impingement is stage I. It is also able to detect subacromial narrowing, fluid pooling in the subacromial or subdeltoid bursae and the presence of joint effusion; all of these are hallmarks of stage I impingement.

The synovitis that accompanies stage II can be detected through a combination of regular ultrasonography and Doppler ultrasonography.

The characteristics of stage III impingement (tendinopathy, tendon tears, effusion, AC joint narrowing) can all be detected accurately using ultrasonography as well. All of this allows for ultrasonography to be used to both diagnose and stage impingement syndrome.

Naredo et al (1999) have suggested that ultrasound can be very helpful in distinguishing differentials from one another, especially between cuff tears and intra-substance tendon pathologies.

Ultrasound can also accurately assess the muscle mass of the rotator cuff muscles especially supraspinatus.

Dynamic ultrasonography is an important tool in properly assessing subacromial impingement, and thereby guiding treatment in an effective and accurate manner. It is able to quickly and cheaply diagnose and stage the disease, as well as determine the likely cause of the problem, providing vital information for both surgeons and physiotherapists. It should be included in the standard tests done to establish whether impingement is present.

Ultrasonography can also be used to guide injections used in shoulder therapy as in calcification of the tendons, and in needle aspiration or lavage of a joint.

CT-scanning is often used following shoulder injuries to assess the damage to the bony structures. It can use reconstructions in multiple planes to assess fractures, measure fragments and determine how severe the damage to the bone has become.

CT-scanning also has an important role to play in the detection and management of dislocations and occult fractures to the shoulder joint, and are integral in the preoperative planning process.

Magnetic resonance imaging is considered the gold standard of shoulder imaging. It clearly shows the anatomy of the shoulder and its pathologies.

Correct use of MRI imaging demands a solid understanding of healthy anatomy, and how MRI images can be interpreted incorrectly.

MRI scans help the physician to distinguish several types of soft tissue and to assess a number of pathologies in a variety of planes. In contrast to ultrasonography, MRI imaging can be used without contrast, and the can accurately assess bursal effusions and hypertrophy.

MRI scan is generally more sensitive and specific than ultrasounds, but they require the highly skilled and specialized musculoskeletal radiologists to get the best possible performance.

Contrast may be used in conjunction with an MRI in order to assess intra-articular bodies and cartilage or labral lesions. Contrast MRI images are also more able to detect sub-surface and partial tears and are better suited to postoperative imaging.

A meta-analysis revealed that the sensitivity and specificity of contrast MRI for rotator cuff lesions are between 80 and 100% (Schulte-Altedorneburg et al, 2003).

Some studies suggested that acromial malformation is a cause of rotator cuff disease, whilst others have suggested it is in fact a consequence. Regardless, narrowing of the subacromial space or tendinous thinning in the region increases one's risk of developing impingement syndrome.

If an MRI (sagittal and frontal view) finds a layer of fat between the supraspinatus and the arch, the patient most likely does not have impingement.

An MRI can also estimate the acromio-humeral distance which is related to the development of tears and impingement if reduced. It is uncommon for the subacromial or subdeltoid bursa to be thicker than 2mm in a healthy adult, though this can change in impingement. As with all other imaging, all changes must be considered in the context of the patient's clinical picture.

MRI has replaced cadaver anatomy as the basis for understanding muscular structures, due to the modality's reliability and fidelity.

MRI scans show that muscle volume is between 1.5 and 1.7 times higher in live humans than in cadavers, most likely do to dehydration after death.

Ultrasonography also provides a reasonably accurate estimate of muscle mass, especially when looking at supraspinatus.

Lehtinen et al (2003) invented a system to reliably measure rotator cuff muscle masses by using MRI scans; in their work, inter-observer and intra-observer variation was less than 4%.

Subscapularis has a volume of 99-165mm^3; infraspinatus and teres minor are 96-125 mm^3 (measured as one due to their indistinct border); supraspinatus is 35-50 mm^3. If a muscle occupies less than half of its respective fossa, it is considered to be atrophied.

MRI can also be used to assess fatty degeneration, using T1-weighted images to classify degeneration according to the Goutallier score (243). Grade 0 is where there is no fat; Grade I is the presence of fatty streaks; Grade II is where muscle occupies more muscle than fat; Grade III is where muscle and fat occupy a similar volume; Grade IV is where fat occupies more space than muscle. Fatty degeneration can have a significant negative impact on the recovery of rotator cuff pathology.

ACKNOWLEDGEMET

The author of this book Dr Sabah Hasan Shindakh would like to express his sincere gratitude for the professors and doctors from the College of Medicine, University of Granada who supervised and evaluated his thesis Dr. Fernando R. Santiago, and Professor Doctor Jose Luis Martin Rodreiguez, Dr Serran Olea Necolas, and assistat professor, Doctor Mariana Fatima Fernandez Cabrera.

Dr Sabah would like also to acknowledge the encouragement and support of his family during the preparation of the thesis and this book.

Dr Sabah didn't forget the help and support of his dear supported Dr. Warjan, and Miss Reem Riyad.

BIBLIOGRAPHY

(1).Brox, J.I. 2003. "Regional musculoskeletal conditions: shoulder pain". Best Practice & Research. Clinical Rheumatology, vol. 17, no. 1, pp. 33-56.

(2).Maffulli, N., Khan, K.M. & Puddu, G. 1998. "Overuse tendon conditions: time to change a confusing terminology". Arthroscopy: The Journal of Arthroscopic & Related Surgery, vol. 14, no. 8, pp. 840-843.

(3).McFarland, E.G., Maffulli, N., Del Buono, A., Murrell, G.A., Garzon-Muvdi, J. & Petersen, S.A. 2013. "Impingement is not impingement: the case for calling it "Rotator Cuff Disease"". Muscles, Ligaments and Tendons Journal, vol. 3, no. 3, pp. 196-200.

(4).Greenberg, D.L. 2014. "Evaluation and treatment of shoulder pain". The Medical Clinics of North America, vol. 98, no. 3, pp. 487-504.

(5).Barr, K.P. 2004. "Rotator cuff disease". Physical Medicine and Rehabilitation Clinics of North America, vol. 15, no. 2, pp. 475-491

(6).Cools, A.M., Cambier, D. & Witvrouw, E.E. 2008. "Screening the athlete's shoulder for impingement symptoms: a clinical reasoning algorithm for early detection of shoulder pathology". British Journal of Sports Medicine, vol. 42, no. 8, pp. 628-635.15).

(6).Bigliani, L.U. & Levine, W.N. 1997. "Subacromial impingement syndrome". The Journal of Bone and Joint Surgery. American volume, vol. 79, no. 12, pp. 1854-1868.

(8).Papadonikolakis, A., McKenna, M., Warme, W., Martin, B.I. & Matsen, F.A., 3rd 2011. "Published evidence relevant to the diagnosis of impingement syndrome of the shoulder". The Journalof Bone and Joint Surgery. American volume, vol. 93, no. 19, pp. 1827-1832.

(9).de Witte, P.B., de Groot, J.H., van Zwet, E.W., Ludewig, P.M., Nagels, J., Nelissen, R.G. & Braman, J.P. 2013. "Communication breakdown: clinicians disagree on subacromial impingement". Medical & Biological Engineering & Computing, vol. 52, no. 3, pp. 221-231.

(10).Palmer, K.T., Harris, E.C., Linaker, C., Cooper, C. & Coggon, D. 2012. "Optimising case definitions of upper limb disorder for aetiological research and prevention: a review". Occupational and Environmental Medicine, vol. 69, no. 1, pp. 71-78.

(11).Neer, C.S., 2nd 1972. "Anterior acromioplasty for the chronic impingement syndrome in the shoulder: a preliminary report". The Journal of Bone and Joint Surgery. American volume, vol. 54, no. 1, pp. 41-50.

(12).Harrison, A.K. & Flatow, E.L. 2011. "Subacromial impingement syndrome". The Journal of the American Academy of Orthopaedic Surgeons, vol. 19, no. 11, pp. 701-708.13).

(13)Goldberg, S.S. & Bigliani, L.U. 2006. "Shoulder impingement revisited: advanced concepts ofpathomechanics and treatment". Instructional Course Lectures, vol. 55, pp. 17-27.

(14)..Goldberg, S.S. & Bigliani, L.U. 2006. "Shoulder impingement revisited: advanced concepts of pathomechanics and treatment". Instructional Course Lectures, vol. 55, pp. 17-27.

(15).Seitz, A.L., McClure, P.W., Finucane, S., Boardman, N.D., 3rd & Michener, L.A. 2011. "Mechanismsof rotator cuff tendinopathy: intrinsic, extrinsic, or both?". Clinical Biomechanics, vol. 26, no. 1, pp. 1-12.

(16).Umer, M., Qadir, I. & Azam, M. 2012. "Subacromial impingement syndrome". Orthopedic Reviews, vol. 4, no. 2, pp. e18.

(17).Morrison, D.S., Bigliani, L.U. & April, E.W. 1987. "The morphology of the acromion and its relationship to rotator cuff tears". Orthop Trans, vol. 11, pp. 439.

(18).Toivonen, D.A., Tuite, M.J. & Orwin, J.F. 1995. "Acromial structure and tears of the rotator cuff". Journal of Shoulder and Elbow Surgery, vol. 4, no. 5, pp. 376-383.

(19).Gagey, N., Ravaud, E. & Lassau, J.P. 1993. "Anatomy of the acromial arch: correlation of anatomy and magnetic resonance imaging". Surgical and Radiologic Anatomy, vol. 15, no. 1, pp. 63- 70.

(20).Gill, T.J., McIrvin, E., Kocher, M.S., Homa, K., Mair, S.D. & Hawkins, R.J. 2002. "The relative importance of acromial morphology and age with respect to rotator cuff pathology". Journal of Shoulder and Elbow Surgery, vol. 11, no. 4, pp. 327-330.

(21).Natsis, K., Tsikaras, P., Totlis, T., Gigis, I., Skandalakis, P., Appell, H.J. & Koebke, J. 2007. "Correlation between the four types of acromion and the existence of enthesophytes: a study on 423 dried scapulas and review of the literature". Clinical Anatomy, vol. 20, no. 3, pp. 267-272.

(.22).Chen, A.L., Rokito, A.S. & Zuckerman, J.D. 2003. "The role of the acromioclavicular joint in impingement syndrome". Clinics in Sports Medicine, vol. 22, no. 2, pp. 343-357.

(23).Cuomo, F., Kummer, F.J., Zuckerman, J.D., Lyon, T., Blair, B. & Olsen, T. 1998. "The influence of acromioclavicular joint morphology on rotator cuff tears". Journal of Shoulder and Elbow Surgery, vol. 7, no. 6, pp. 555-559.

(24).Neer, C.S., 2nd 1983. "Impingement lesions". Clinical Orthopaedics and Related Research, vol. (173), no. 173, pp. 70-77.

(.25).Kesmezacar, H., Akgun, I., Ogut, T., Gokay, S. & Uzun, I. 2008. "The coracoacromial ligament: the morphology and relation to rotator cuff pathology". Journal of Shoulder and Elbow Surgery, vol. 17, no. 1, pp. 182-188.

(26).Wright, R.W., Heller, M.A., Quick, D.C. & Buss, D.D. 2000. "Arthroscopic decompression for impingement syndrome secondary to an unstable os acromiale". Arthroscopy: The Journal of Arthroscopic & Related Surgery, vol. 16, no. 6, pp. 595-599.

(27).Boehm, T.D., Matzer, M., Brazda, D. & Gohlke, F.E. 2003. "Os acromiale associated with tear of the rotator cuff treated operatively. Review of 33 patients". The Journal of Bone and Joint Surgery. British volume, vol. 85, no. 4, pp. 545-549.

(28)Boehm, T.D., Rolf, O., Martetschlaeger, F., Kenn, W. & Gohlke, F. 2005. "Rotator cuff tears associated with os acromiale". Acta Orthopaedica, vol. 76, no. 2, pp. 241-244.

(29).Ferrick, M.R. 2000. "Coracoid impingement. A case report and review of the literature". The American Journal of Sports Medicine, vol. 28, no. 1, pp. 117-119.

(30).Lo, I.K., Parten, P.M. & Burkhart, S.S. 2003. "Combined subcoracoid and subacromial impingement in association with anterosuperior rotator cuff tears: An arthroscopic approach". Arthroscopy: The Journal of Arthroscopic & Related Surgery, vol. 19, no. 10, pp. 1068-1078.

(31).Richards, D.P., Burkhart, S.S. & Campbell, S.E. 2005. "Relation between narrowed coracohumeral distance and subscapularis tears". Arthroscopy: The Journal of Arthroscopic & Related Surgery, vol. 21, no. 10, pp. 1223-1228.

(32).Osti, L., Soldati, F., Del Buono, A. & Massari, L. 2013. "Subcoracoid impingement and subscapularis tendon: is there any truth?".Muscles, Ligaments and Tendons Journal, vol. 3, no. 2, pp. 101- 105.

(33).Harvie, P., Ostlere, S.J., Teh, J., McNally, E.G., Clipsham, K., Burston, B.J., Pollard, T.C. & Carr, A.J. 2004. "Genetic influences in the aetiology of tears of the rotator cuff. Sibling risk of a full-thickness tear". The Journal of Bone and Joint Surgery. British volume, vol. 86, no. 5, pp. 696-700.

(34).Obaid, H. & Connell, D. 2010. "Cell therapy in tendon disorders: what is the current evidence?". The American Journal of Sports Medicine, vol. 38, no. 10, pp. 2123-2132.

(35).Miranda, H., Viikari-Juntura, E., Martikainen, R., Takala, E.P. & Riihimaki, H. 2001. "A prospective study of work related factors and physical exercise as predictors of shoulder pain". Occupational and Environmental Medicine, vol. 58, no. 8, pp. 528-534.

(36).Neviaser, A., Andarawis-Puri, N. & Flatow, E. 2012. "Basic mechanisms of tendon fatigue damage". Journal of Shoulder and Elbow Surgery, vol. 21, no. 2, pp. 158-163.

(37).Andres, B.M. & Murrell, G.A. 2008. "Treatment of tendinopathy: what works, what does not, and what is on the horizon". Clinical Orthopaedics and Related Research, vol. 466, no. 7, pp. 1539-1554.

(38).Castagna, A., Garofalo, R., Cesari, E., Marcopoulos, N., Borroni, M. & Conti, M. 2010. "Anterior and posterior internal impingement: an evidence-based review". British Journal of Sports Medicine, vol. 44, no. 5, pp. 382-388

(39).Kirchhoff, C. & Imhoff, A.B. 2010. "Posterosuperior and anterosuperior impingement of the shoulder in overhead athletes-evolving concepts". International Orthopaedics, vol. 34, no.
7, pp. 1049-1058.

(40).Jobe, C.M. & Iannotti, J.P. 1995. "Limits imposed on glenohumeral motion by joint geometry". Journal of Shoulder and Elbow Surgery, vol. 4, no. 4, pp. 281-285.

(41).Paley, K.J., Jobe, F.W., Pink, M.M., Kvitne, R.S. & El Attrache, N.S. 2000. "Arthroscopic findings in the overhand throwing athlete: evidence for posterior internal impingement of the rotator cuff". Arthroscopy: The Journal of Arthroscopic & Related Surgery, vol. 16, no. 1, pp. 35-4.

(42).Manske, R.C., Grant-Nierman, M. & Lucas, B. 2013. "Shoulder posterior internal impingement in the overhead athlete". International Journal of Sports Physical Therapy, vol. 8, no. 2, pp. 194-204.

(43).Michener, L.A., McClure, P.W. & Karduna, A.R. 2003. "Anatomical and biomechanical mechanisms of subacromial impingement syndrome". Clinical Biomechanics, vol. 18, no. 5,
pp. 369-379

(44).Bodin, J., Ha, C., Chastang, J.F., Descatha, A., Leclerc, A., Goldberg, M., Imbernon, E. & Roquelaure, Y. 2012. "Comparison of risk factors for shoulder pain and rotator cuff
syndrome in the working population". American Journal of Industrial Medicine, vol. 55, no.
7, pp. 605-615

(45).Bonsell, S., Pearsall, A.W., 4th, Heitman, R.J., Helms, C.A., Major, N.M. & Speer, K.P. 2000. "The relationship of age, gender, and degenerative changes observed on radiographs of the shoulder in asymptomatic individuals". The Journal of Bone and Joint Surgery. British volume, vol. 82, no. 8, pp. 1135-1139

(46).Buckle, P. 1997. "Upper limb disorders and work: the importance of physical and psychosocial factors". Journal of Psychosomatic Research, vol. 43, no. 1, pp. 17-25

(47).Miranda, H., Viikari-Juntura, E., Heistaro, S., Heliovaara, M. & Riihimaki, H. 2005. "A population study on differences in the determinants of a specific shoulder disorder versus nonspecific -shoulder pain without clinical findings". American Journal of Epidemiology, vol. 161, no. 9, pp. 847-855.

(48).Rechardt, M., Shiri, R., Karppinen, J., Jula, A., Heliovaara, M. & Viikari-Juntura, E. 2010. "Lifestyle and metabolic factors in relation to shoulder pain and rotator cuff tendinitis: a population based study". BMC Musculoskeletal Disorders, vol. 11, pp. 165.

(49).Roquelaure, Y., Bodin, J., Ha, C., Petit Le Manac'h, A., Descatha, A., Chastang, J.F., Leclerc,A., Goldberg, M. & Imbernon, E. 2011. "Personal, biomechanical, and psychosocial risk factors for rotator cuff syndrome in a working population". Scandinavian Journal of Work, Environment & Health, vol. 37, no. 6, pp. 502-511.

(50).Moosmayer, S. & Smith, H.J. 2005. "Diagnostic ultrasound of the shoulder – a method for experts only? Results from an orthopedic surgeon with relative inexpensive compared to operative findings". Acta Orthopaedica, vol. 76, no. 4, pp. 503-508.

(51).Nove-Josserand, L., Walch, G., Adeleine, P. & Courpron, P. 2005. "Effect of age on the naturalhistory of the shoulder: a clinical and radiological study in the elderly". Revue de Chirurgie Orthopedique et Reparatrice de l'appareil Moteur, vol. 91, no. 6, pp. 508-514

(52).Yamaguchi, K., Ditsios, K., Middleton, W.D., Hildebolt, C.F., Galatz, L.M. & Teefey, S.A. 2006. "The demographic and morphological features of rotator cuff disease. A comparison of asymptomatic and symptomatic shoulders". The Journal of Bone and Joint Surgery. Americanvolume, vol. 88, no. 8, pp. 1699-1704.

(53).Yamamoto, A., Takagishi, K., Osawa, T., Yanagawa, T., Nakajima, D., Shitara, H. & Kobayashi, T. 2010. "Prevalence and risk factors of a rotator cuff tear in the general population". Journal of Shoulder and Elbow Surgery, vol. 19, no. 1, pp. 116-120.

(54).Yamaguchi, K., Tetro, A.M., Blam, O., Evanoff, B.A., Teefey, S.A. & Middleton, W.D. 2001. "Natural history of asymptomatic rotator cuff tears: a longitudinal analysis of asymptomatic tears detected sonographically". Journal of Shoulder and Elbow Surgery, vol. 10, no. 3, pp. 199-203.

(55).Chang, W.K. 2004. "Shoulder impingement syndrome". Physical Medicine and Rehabilitation Clinics of North America, vol. 15, no. 2, pp. 493-510.

(56).Wang, J.C. & Shapiro, M.S. 1997. "Changes in acromial morphology with age". Journal of Shoulder and Elbow Surgery, vol. 6, no. 1, pp. 55-59.

(57).Tekavec, E., Joud, A., Rittner, R., Mikoczy, Z., Nordander, C., Petersson, I.F. & Englund, M. 2012. "Population-based consultation patterns in patients with shoulder pain diagnoses". BMC Musculoskeletal Disorders, vol. 13, pp. 238.

(58)., J.P., Mikkelsen, S., Andersen, J.H., Fallentin, N., Baelum, J., Svendsen, S.W., Thomsen, J.F., Frost, P., Thomsen, G., Overgaard, E., Kaergaard, A. & PRIM Health Study Group 2003. "Prognosis of shoulder tendonitis in repetitive work: a follow up study in a cohort of Danish industrial and service workers". Occupational and Environmental Medicine, vol. 60, no. 9, pp. E8.

(59).Wijnhoven, H.A., de Vet, H.C. & Picavet, H.S. 2006. "Explaining sex differences in chronic musculoskeletal pain in a general population". Pain, vol. 124, no. 1-2, pp. 158-166.

(60).Eltayeb, S., Staal, J.B., Kennes, J., Lamberts, P.H. & de Bie, R.A. 2007. "Prevalence of complaints of arm, neck and shoulder among computer office workers and psychometric evaluation of a risk factor questionnaire". BMC Musculoskeletal Disorders, vol. 8, pp. 68 .

(61).Bot, S.D., van der Waal, J.M., Terwee, C.B., van der Windt, D.A., Schellevis, F.G., Bouter, L.M. & Dekker, J. 2005a. "Incidence and prevalence of complaints of the neck and upper extremity in general practice". Annals of the Rheumatic Diseases, vol. 64, no. 1, pp. 118-123.

(62).Wofford, J.L., Mansfield, R.J. & Watkins, R.S. 2005. "Patient characteristics and clinical management of patients with shoulder pain in

U.S. primary care settings: secondary dataanalysis of the National Ambulatory Medical Care Survey". BMC Musculoskeletal Disorders, vol. 6, pp. 4.

(63).Linsell, L., Dawson, J., Zondervan, K., Rose, P., Randall, T., Fitzpatrick, R. & Carr, A. 2006. "Prevalence and incidence of adults consulting for shoulder conditions in UK primary care; patterns of diagnosis and referral". Rheumatology (Oxford, England), vol. 45, no. 2, pp. 215-221 .

(64).www.terveys2000.fi/julkaisut) .

(65).Silverstein, B.A., Viikari-Juntura, E., Fan, Z.J., Bonauto, D.K., Bao, S. & Smith, C. 2006. "Natural course of nontraumatic rotator cuff tendinitis and shoulder symptoms in a working population". Scandinavian Journal of Work, Environment & Health, vol. 32, no. 2, pp. 99-108.

(66).Roquelaure, Y., Ha, C., Rouillon, C., Fouquet, N., Leclerc, A., Descatha, A., Touranchet, A., Goldberg, M., Imbernon, E. & Members of Occupational Health Services of the Pays de la Loire Region 2009. "Risk factors for upper-extremity musculoskeletal disorders in the working population". Arthritis and Rheumatism, vol. 61, no. 10, pp. 1425-1434.

(67).van Rijn, R.M., Huisstede, B.M., Koes, B.W. & Burdorf, A. 2010. "Associations between work related factors and specific disorders of the shoulder – a systematic review of the literature". Scandinavian Journal of Work, Environment & Health, vol. 36, no. 3, pp. 189-201.

(68).Bodin, J., Ha, C., Petit, A., Descatha, A., Thomas, T., Goldberg, M., Leclerc, A. & Roquelaure, Y. 2014. "Natural course of rotator cuff syndrome in a French working population". American Journal of Industrial Medicine, vol. 57, no. 6, pp. 683-694.

(69).Frost, P. & Andersen, J.H. 1999. "Shoulder impingement syndrome in relation to shoulder intensive work". Occupational and Environmental Medicine, vol. 56, no. 7, pp. 494-498.

(70).Makela, M., Heliovaara, M., Sainio, P., Knekt, P., Impivaara, O. & Aromaa, A. 1999. "Shoulder joint impairment among Finns aged 30 years or over: prevalence, risk factors and co-morbidity". Rheumatology, vol. 38, no. 7, pp. 656-662.

(71).Bonde, J.P., Mikkelsen, S., Andersen, J.H., Fallentin, N., Baelum, J., Svendsen, S.W., Thomsen, J.F., Frost, P., Thomsen, G., Overgaard, E., Kaergaard, A. & PRIM Health Study Group 2003. "Prognosis of shoulder tendonitis in repetitive work: a follow up study in a cohort of Danish industrial and service workers". Occupational and Environmental Medicine, vol. 60, no. 9, pp. E8.

(72).Reilingh, M.L., Kuijpers, T., Tanja-Harfterkamp, A.M. & van der Windt, D.A. 2008. "Course and prognosis of shoulder symptoms in general practice". Rheumatology, vol. 47, no.5, pp. 108. 724-730.

(73).Macfarlane, G.J., Norrie, G., Atherton, K., Power, C. & Jones, G.T. 2009. "The influence of socioeconomic status on the reporting of regional and widespread musculoskeletal pain: results from the 1958 British Birth Cohort Study". Annals of the Rheumatic Diseases, vol. 68, no. 10, pp. 1591-1595.

(74).Bot, S.D., van der Waal, J.M., Terwee, C.B., van der Windt, D.A., Scholten, R.J., Bouter, L.M. & Dekker, J. 2005b. "Predictors of outcome in neck and shoulder symptoms: a cohort study in general practice". Spine, vol. 30, no. 16, pp. E459-470.

(75).Chipchase, L.S., O'Connor, D.A., Costi, J.J. & Krishnan, J. 2000. "Shoulder impingement syndrome: preoperative health status". Journal of Shoulder and Elbow Surgery, vol. 9, no. 1, pp. 12-15.

(76).George, S.Z., Wallace, M.R., Wright, T.W., Moser, M.W., Greenfield, W.H., 3rd, Sack, B.K., Herbstman, D.M. & Fillingim, R.B. 2008. "Evidence for a biopsychosocial influence on shoulder pain: pain catastrophizing and catechol-O-methyltransferase (COMT) diplotype predict clinical pain ratings". Pain, vol. 136, no. 1-2, pp. 53-61.

(77).Luime, J.J., Kuiper, J.I., Koes, B.W., Verhaar, J.A., Miedema, H.S. & Burdorf, A. 2004. "Workrelated risk factors for the incidence and recurrence of shoulder and neck complaints among nursing-home and elderly-care workers". Scandinavian Journal of Work, Environment &Health, vol. 30, no. 4, pp. 279-286.

(78).Wendelboe, A.M., Hegmann, K.T., Gren, L.H., Alder, S.C., White, G.L., Jr & Lyon, J.L. 2004. "Associations between body-mass index and surgery for rotator cuff tendinitis". The Journalof Bone and Joint Surgery. American volume, vol. 86-A, no. 4, pp. 743-747.

(79).Gomoll, A.H., Katz, J.N., Warner, J.J. & Millett, P.J. 2004. "Rotator cuff disorders: recognition and management among patients with shoulder pain". Arthritis and Rheumatism, vol. 50, no. 12, pp. 3751-3761.

(80).Andrews, J.R. 2005. "Diagnosis and treatment of chronic painful shoulder: review of nonsurgical interventions". Arthroscopy: The Journal of Arthroscopic & Related Surgery, vol. 21, no. 3, pp.
333-347.

(81).Mulligan, E.P., Brunette, M., Shirley, Z. & Khazzam, M. 2015. "Sleep quality and nocturnal pain in patients with shoulder disorders". Journal of shoulder and elbow surgery, vol. 24, no. 9, pp. 1452-1457

(82).Koester, M.C., George, M.S. & Kuhn, J.E. 2005. "Shoulder impingement syndrome". The American Journal of Medicine, vol. 118, no. 5, pp. 452-455.

(83).van der Heijden, G.J. 1999. "Shoulder disorders: a state-of-the-art review". Bailliere's Best Practice & Research. Clinical Rheumatology, vol. 13, no. 2, pp. 287-309.

(84).Goldstein, B. 2004. "Shoulder anatomy and biomechanics". Physical Medicine and Rehabilitation Clinics of North America, vol. 15, no. 2, pp. 313-349

(85).Schultz, J.S. 2004. "Clinical evaluation of the shoulder". Physical Medicine and Rehabilitation Clinics of North America, vol. 15, no. 2, pp. 351-371.

(86).Yamamoto, N., Muraki, T., Sperling, J.W., Steinmann, S.P., Itoi, E., Cofield, R.H. &An, K.N. 2009. "Impingement mechanisms of the Neer and Hawkins signs". Journal of Shoulder andElbow Surgery, vol. 18, no. 6, pp. 942-947.

(87).Calis, M., Akgun, K., Birtane, M., Karacan, I., Calis, H. & Tuzun, F. 2000. "Diagnostic values of clinical diagnostic tests in subacromial impingement syndrome". Annals of the RheumaticDiseases, vol. 59, no. 1, pp. 44-47.

(88).MacDonald, P.B., Clark, P. & Sutherland, K. 2000. "An analysis of the diagnostic accuracy of the Hawkins and Neer subacromial impingement signs". Journal of Shoulder and Elbow Surgery, vol. 9, no. 4, pp. 299-301.

(89).Hanchard, N.C., Lenza, M., Handoll, H.H. & Takwoingi, Y. 2013. "Physical tests for shoulder impingements and local lesions of bursa, tendon or labrum that may accompany impingement". The Cochrane Database of Systematic Reviews, vol. 4, pp. CD007427.

(90).van Kampen, D.A., van den Berg, T., van der Woude, H.J., Castelein, R.M., Scholtes, V.A., Terwee, C.B. & Willems, W.J. 2014. "The diagnostic value of the combination of patient characteristics, history, and clinical shoulder tests for the diagnosis of rotator cuff tear". Journal of Orthopaedic Surgery and Research, vol. 9, pp. 70.

(91).Hawkins, R.J. & Kennedy, J.C. 1980. "Impingement syndrome in athletes". The American Journal of Sports Medicine, vol. 8, no. 3, pp. 151-158.

(92).Leroux, J.L., Thomas, E., Bonnel, F. & Blotman, F. 1995. "Diagnostic value of clinical tests for shoulder impingement syndrome". Revue du Rhumatisme (English ed.), vol. 62, no. 6, pp. 423-428.

(93).Hertel, R., Ballmer, F.T., Lombert, S.M. & Gerber, C. 1996. "Lag signs in the diagnosis of rotator cuff rupture". Journal of Shoulder and Elbow Surgery, vol. 5, no. 4, pp. 307-313.

(94).Gerber, C., Hersche, O. & Farron, A. 1996. "Isolated rupture of the subscapularis tendon". The Journal of Bone and Joint Surgery. American volume, vol. 78, no. 7, pp. 1015-1023.

(95).Hermans, J., Luime, J.J., Meuffels, D.E., Reijman, M., Simel, D.L. & Bierma-Zeinstra, S.M. 2013. "Does this patient with shoulder pain have rotator cuff disease?: The Rational Clinical Examination systematic review". JAMA: the Journal of the American Medical Association, vol. 310, no. 8, pp. 837-847.

(96).Park, H.B., Yokota, A., Gill, H.S., El Rassi, G. & McFarland, E.G. 2005. "Diagnostic accuracy of clinical tests for the different degrees of subacromial impingement syndrome". The Journalof Bone and Joint Surgery. American volume, vol. 87, no. 7, pp. 1446-1455.

(97).Diercks, R., Bron, C., Dorrestijn, O., Meskers, C., Naber, R., de Ruiter, T., Willems, J., Winters, J., van der Woude, H.J. & Dutch Orthopaedic Association 2014. "Guideline for diagnosis and treatment of subacromial pain syndrome: a multidisciplinary review by the Dutch Orthopaedic Association". Acta Orthopaedica, vol. 85, no. 3, pp. 314-322.

(98). Heyworth B, Williams R. Internal Impingement of the Shoulder. The American Journal of Sports Medicine. (2009) 37:1024-1037, Level of Evidence: 2A

(99). Behrens S, Compas J, Deren M, Drakos M. Internal Impingement: A Review on a Common Cause of Shoulder Pain in Throwers. The Physician and Sportsmedicine. (2010) 38:2, Level of Evidence: 2A.

(100). Drakos M, Rudzki J, Allen A, Potter H, Altchek D. Internal Impingement of the Shoulder in the Overhead Athlete. Journal of Bone; Joint Surgery. (2009) 91:2719-2718, Level of Evidence: 2A
(101). Jobe C, Coen M, Screnar P. Evaluation of Impingement Syndromes in the Overhead-Throwing Athlete. Journal of Athletic Training. (2000) 35:293-299, Level of Evidence 3A.

(102) Hanchard NC, Lenza M, Handoll HH, Takwoingi Y. Physical tests for shoulder impingements and local lesions of bursa, tendon or labrum that may accompany impingement. Cochrane Database Syst Rev. 2013 Apr

(103).Chard, M.D., Hazleman, R., Hazleman, B.L., King, R.H. & Reiss, B.B. 1991. "Shoulder disorders in the elderly: a community survey". Arthritis and Rheumatism, vol. 34, no. 6, pp. 766-76.

(104).Green, S., Buchbinder, R. & Hetrick, S. 2003. "Physiotherapy interventions for shoulder pain". Cochrane Database of Systematic Reviews, vol. (2), no. 2, pp. CD004258.

(105).Greving, K., Dorrestijn, O., Winters, J.C., Groenhof, F., van der Meer, K., Stevens, M. & Diercks, R.L. 2012. "Incidence, prevalence, and consultation rates of shoulder complaints in general practice". Scandinavian Journal of Rheumatology, vol. 41, no. 2, pp. 150-155.

(106).Picavet, H.S. & Schouten, J.S. 2003. "Musculoskeletal pain in the Netherlands: prevalences, consequences and risk groups, the DMC(3)-study". Pain, vol. 102, no. 1-2, pp. 167-178.

(107).Urwin, M., Symmons, D., Allison, T., Brammah, T., Busby, H., Roxby, M., Simmons, A. & Williams, G. 1998. "Estimating the burden of musculoskeletal disorders in the community: the comparative prevalence of symptoms at different anatomical sites, and the relation to social deprivation". Annals of the Rheumatic Diseases, vol. 57, no. 11, pp. 649-655.

(108).van der Windt, D.A., Koes, B.W., de Jong, B.A. & Bouter, L.M. 1995. "Shoulder disorders in general practice: incidence, patient characteristics, and management". Annals of the Rheumatic Diseases, vol. 54, no. 12, pp. 959-964.

(109).van der Windt, D.A., Koes, B.W., Boeke, A.J., Deville, W., De Jong, B.A. & Bouter, L.M. 1996. "Shoulder disorders in general practice: prognostic indicators of outcome". The BritishJournal of General Practice, vol. 46, no. 410, pp. 519-523.

(110).Vecchio, P., Kavanagh, R., Hazleman, B.L. & King, R.H. 1995. "Shoulder pain in a community based rheumatology clinic". British Journal of Rheumatology, vol. 34, no. 5, pp. 440-442.

(111).Luime, J.J., Koes, B.W., Hendriksen, I.J., Burdorf, A., Verhagen, A.P., Miedema, H.S. & Verhaar, J.A. 2004. "Prevalence and incidence of shoulder pain in the general population; a systematic

(112). Gray H. The humerus. In: Gray H, editor. Anatomy of the humanbody. Philadelphia: Lea & Febiger; 1918. Scandinavian Journal of Rheumatology, vol. 33, no. 2, pp. 73-81.

(113).Morag Y, Jacobson JA, Shields G, Rajani R, Jamadar DA, Miller B, et al. MR arthrog-raphy of rotator interval, long head of the biceps brachii, and biceps pulley ofthe shoulder. Radiology2005;235(1):21–30.

(114) Bureau NJ, Dussault RG, Keats TE. Imaging of bursae around the shoulder joint.Skelet Radiol 1996;25(6):513–7.

(115) Ha AS, Petscavage-Thomas JM, Tagoylo GH. Acromioclavicular joint: the other joint in the shoulder. AJR Am J Roentgenol 2014;202(2):375–85.

.(116). Epstein D, Day M, Rokito A. Current concepts in the surgical manage-ment of acromioclavicular joint injuries. Bull NYU Hosp Jt Dis 2012;70(1):11–24.

(117). Minagawa H, Itoi E, Konno N, Kido T, Sano A, Uramaya M, et al. Humeral attachment of the supraspinatus and infraspinatus tendons: an anatomic study.Arthroscopy 1998;14(3):302–6.

.(118). Ruotolo C, Fow JE, Nottage WM. The supraspinatus footprint: an anatomic studyof the supraspinatus insertion. Arthroscopy 2004;20(3):246–9 487-91.

(119). Crass JR, Craig EV, Thompson RC, Feinberg SB. Ultrasonography of the rotator cuff: surgical correlation. J Clin Ultrasound 1984; 12.

(121). Rockwood Jr CA, Jensen KL. X-ray evaluation of shoulder problems. In: Rockwood Jr CA, Matsen III FA, Wirth MA, Harryman DT, eds. The Shoulder. 2nd ed. Philadelphia: WB Saunders; 1998:199-231.

(122). Goud A, Segal D, Hedayati P, Pan JJ, Weissman BN. Radiographic evaluation of the shoulder. Eur J Radiol 2008;68:2-15.

(123). Blaine TA, Bigliani LU, Levine WN. Fractures of the proximal humerus. In: Rockwood Jr CA, Matsen III FA, Wirth MA, Harryman DT, eds. The Shoulder. 3rd ed. Philadelphia: WB Saunders; 2004.p.355-412.

(124). Magee DJ. Ortopedic physical assessment. 3rd edition. Philadelphia: WB Saunders; 1997.pp.175-246.

(125). Bigliani LU, Ticker JB, Flatow EL, Soslowsky LJ, Mow VC. The relationship of acromial architecture to rotator cuff disease. Clin Sports Med 1991;10:823-38.

(126). Weiner DS, Macnab I. Superior migration of the humeral head. A radiological aid in the diagnosis of tears of the rotator cuff. J Bone Joint Surg Br 1970;52:524-7.

(127). Rubin SA, Gray RL, Green WR. The scapular "Y": a diagnostic aid in shoulder trauma. Radiology 1974;110:725-6.

(128) . Martinoli C , Bianchi S , Prato N , et al . US of the shoulder: non-rotator cuff disorders . Radio-Graphics 2003 ; 23 (2): 381-401 ; quiz 534 .

(129) . Moosikasuwan JB , Miller TT , Burke BJ . Rotator cuff tears: clinical, radiographic, and US findings . Radio Graphics 2005 ; 25 (6): 1591 -1607.

(130) . Teefey SA , Hasan SA , Middleton WD , Patel M , Wright RW , Yamaguchi K . Ultrasonography of the rotator cuff: a comparison of ultrasonographic and arthroscopic fi ndings in one hundred consecutive cases . J Bone Joint Surg Am 2000 ; 82 (4): 498 – 504.

(131) . Vlychou M , Dailiana Z , Fotiadou A , Papanagiotou M , Fezoulidis IV , Malizos K .Symptomatic partial rotator cuff tears: diagnostic performance of ultrasound and magnetic resonance imaging with surgical correlation . Acta Radiol 2009 ; 50 (1): 101 – 105.

(132) . Le Corroller T , Cohen M , Aswad R , Pauly V , Champsaur P . Sonography of the painful shoulder: role of the operator's experience .Skeletal Radiol 2008 ; 37 (11): 979 – 986 .

(133) . Jamadar DA , Jacobson JA , Caoili EM , et al . Musculoskeletal sonography technique: focused versus comprehensive evaluation . AJR Am J Roentgenol 2008 ; 190 (1): 5-9.

(134) . Crass JR , Craig EV , Feinberg SB . The hyperextended internal rotation view in rotator cuff ultrasonography . J Clin Ultrasound 1987 ; 15 (6): 416 – 420 .

(135) . Ferri M , Finlay K , Popowich T , Stamp G ,Schuringa P , Friedman L . Sonography of full-thickness supraspinatus tears: comparison of patient positioning technique with surgical correlation . AJR Am J Roentgenol 2005 ; 184 (1): 180 – 184.

(136) . Bureau NJ , Beauchamp M , Cardinal E , Brassard P . Dynamic sonography evaluation of shoulder impingement syndrome . AJR Am J Roentgenol 2006 ; 187 (1): 216 – 220 .

(137) . Morag Y , Jacobson JA , Miller B , De Maeseneer M , Girish G , Jamadar D . MR imaging of rotator cuff injury: what the clinician needs to know . RadioGraphics 2006 ; 26 (4): 1045 – 1065.

(138) . Khoury V , Cardinal E , Brassard P . Atrophy and fatty infiltration of the supraspinatus muscle: sonography versus MRI . AJR Am J Roentgenol 2008 ; 190 (4): 1105 – 1111 .

(139).Garner, Hillary Warren. "Problem Solving in Musculoskeletal Imaging." American Journal of Roentgenology 193.1 (2009): W72-W72

(140). Coumas J, Waite R, Goss T, Ferrari DA, Kanzaria PK, Pappas AM. CT and MR evaluation of the labral capsular ligamentous complex of the shoulder. AJR Am J Roentgenol 1992;158:591-7.

(141). Baudi P, Righi P, Bolognesi D, Rivetta S, Rossi Urtoler E, Guicciardi N, et al. How to identify and calculate glenoid bone deficit. Chir Organi Mov 2005;90:145-52.

(142). Magarelli N, Milano G, Sergio P, Santagada DA, Fabbriciani C, Bonomo L. Intra-observer and interobserver reliability of the 'Pico' computed tomography method for quantification of glenoid bone defect in anterior shoulder instability. Skeletal Radiol 2009;38:1071-5.

(143).ACRSSR Practice Guideline for the Performance and Interpretation of Magnetic Resonance Imaging (MRI) of the Shoulder. American College of Radiology (ACR). Reston, Virginia,USA 2010. (http://www.acr.org/~/media/ACR/Documents/PGTS/guidelines/MRI_Shoulder.pdf).

(144). Modarresi S, Jude CM. Radiologic evaluation of the painful shoulder 2012 UpTo Date. Available from: URL: www.uptodate.com.

(145) . De Maeseneer M, Van Roy F, Lenchik L, Shahabpour M, Jacobson J, Ryu KN, et al. CT and MR arthrography of the normal and pathologic anterosuperior labrum and labral-bicipital complex. Radiographics 2000;20:67-81.

(146). Goutallier D, Postel JM, Bernageau J, Lavau L, Voisin MC. Fatty muscle degeneration in cuff ruptures. Pre- and postoperative evaluation by CT scan. Clin Orthop Relat Res 1994;304:78-83.

(147). Fuchs B, Weishaupt D, Zanetti M, Hodler J, Gerber C. Fatty degeneration of the muscles of the rotator cuff: assessment by computed tomography versus magnetic resonance imaging. J Shoulder Elbow Surg 1999;8:599-605.

(148). Oh JH, Kim SH, Choi JA, Kim Y, Oh CH. Reliability of the grading system for fatty degeneration of rotator cuff muscles. Clin Orthop Relat Res 2010;468:1558-64.

(149). Slabaugh MA, Friel NA, Karas V, Romeo AA, Verma NN, Cole BJ. Interobserver and intraobserver reliability of the Goutallier classification using magnetic resonance imaging: proposal of a simplified classification system to increase reliability. Am J Sports Med 2012;40:1728-34.

(150). Alyas F, Curtis M, Speed C, Saifuddin A, Connell D. MR imaging appearances of acromioclavicular joint dislocation. Radiographics 2008;28:463-79.

(151). de la Puente R, Boutin RD, Theodorou DJ, Hooper A, Schweitzer M, Resnick D. Post-traumatic and stress-induced osteolysis of thedistal clavicle: MR imaging findings in 17 patients. Skeletal Radiol 1999;28:202-8.

(152). Shellock FG. Reference manual for magnetic resonance safety. Salt Lake City: Amirsys, Inc ; 2003.

(153). Johansson, K., Oberg, B., Adolfsson, L. & Foldevi, M. 2002. "A combination of systematic review and clinicians' beliefs in interventions for subacromial pain". The British Journal of GeneralPractice, vol. 52, no. 475, pp. 145-152.
(154). Morrison, D.S., Greenbaum, B.S. & Einhorn, A. 2000. "Shoulder impingement". The Orthopedic Clinics of North America, vol. 31, no. 2, pp. 285-293.

(155). van der Windt, D.A., van der Heijden, G.J., Scholten, R.J., Koes, B.W. & Bouter, L.M. 1995. "The efficacy of non-steroidal anti-inflammatory drugs (NSAIDS) for shoulder complaints. A systematic review". Journal of clinical epidemiology, vol. 48, no. 5, pp. 691-704.

(156). Petri, M., Hufman, S.L., Waser, G., Cui, H., Snabes, M.C. & Verburg, K.M. 2004. "Celecoxib effectively treats patients with acute shoulder tendinitis/bursitis". The Journal of Rheumatology, vol. 31, no. 8, pp. 1614-1620.

(157). Min, K.S., St Pierre, P., Ryan, P.M., Marchant, B.G., Wilson, C.J. & Arrington, E.D. 2013. "A double-blind randomized controlled trial comparing the effects of subacromial injection with corticosteroid versus NSAID in patients with shoulder impingement syndrome". Journal of Shoulder and Elbow Surgery, vol. 22, no. 5, pp. 595-601.

(158).Akgun, K., Birtane, M. & Akarirmak, U. 2004. "Is local subacromial corticosteroid injection beneficial in subacromial impingement syndrome?".Clinical Rheumatology, vol. 23, no. 6, pp. 496-500.

(159). Hsieh, L.F., Hsu, W.C., Lin, Y.J., Wu, S.H., Chang, K.C. & Chang, H.L. 2013. "Is ultrasoundguided injection more effective in chronic subacromial bursitis?".Medicine and Science inSports and Exercise, vol. 45, no. 12, pp. 2205-2213.

(160).Gaujoux-Viala, C., Dougados, M. & Gossec, L. 2009. "Efficacy and safety of steroid injections for shoulder and elbow tendonitis: a meta-analysis of randomised controlled trials". Annals ofthe Rheumatic Diseases, vol. 68, no. 12, pp. 1843-1849.

(161). Mitchell, C., Adebajo, A., Hay, E. & Carr, A. 2005. "Shoulder pain: diagnosis and management in primary care". BMJ, vol. 331, no. 7525, pp. 1124-1128.

(162).Dorrestijn, O., Stevens, M., Winters, J.C., van der Meer, K. & Diercks, R.L. 2009. "Conservative or surgical treatment for subacromial impingement syndrome? A systematic review". Journalof Shoulder and Elbow Surgery, vol. 18, no. 4, pp. 652-660.

(163).Chaudhury, S., Gwilym, S.E., Moser, J. & Carr, A.J. 2010. "Surgical options for patients with shoulder pain". Nature Reviews. Rheumatology, vol. 6, no. 4, pp. 217-226.

(164). Gartsman, G.M. 1995. "Arthroscopic treatment of rotator cuff disease". Journal of Shoulder and Elbow Surgery, vol. 4, no. 3, pp. 228-241.

(165). Michener, L.A., Walsworth, M.K. & Burnet, E.N. 2004. "Effectiveness of rehabilitation for patients with subacromial impingement syndrome: a systematic review". Journal of Hand Therapy, vol. 17, no. 2, pp. 152-164.

(166). Senbursa, G., Baltaci, G. & Atay, A. 2007. "Comparison of conservative treatment with and without manual physical therapy for patients with shoulder impingement syndrome: a prospective, randomized clinical trial". Knee Surgery, Sports Traumatology, Arthroscopy, vol. 15, no. 7, pp. 915-921.

(167) Kachingwe, A.F., Phillips, B., Sletten, E. & Plunkett, S.W. 2008. "Comparison of manual therapy techniques with therapeutic exercise in the treatment of shoulder impingement: a randomized controlled pilot clinical trial". The Journal of Manual & Manipulative Therapy, vol. 16, no. 4, pp. 238-247.

(168). Bennell, K., Wee, E., Coburn, S., Green, S., Harris, A., Staples, M., Forbes, A. & Buchbinder, R. 2010. "Efficacy of standardised manual therapy and home exercise programme for chronic rotator cuff disease: randomised placebo controlled trial". BMJ, vol. 340, pp. c2756.

(169). Osteras, H., Torstensen, T.A., Haugerud, L. & Osteras, B.S. 2009. "Dose-response effects of graded therapeutic exercises in patients with long-standing subacromial pain". Advances inPhysiotherapy, vol. 11, pp. 199-209.

(170). Kuhn, J.E. 2009. "Exercise in the treatment of rotator cuff impingement: a systematic review and a synthesized evidence-based rehabilitation protocol". Journal of Shoulder and Elbow Surgery, vol. 18, no. 1, pp. 138-160.

(171). Hanratty, C.E., McVeigh, J.G., Kerr, D.P., Basford, J.R., Finch, M.B., Pendleton, A. & Sim, J. 2012. "The effectiveness of physiotherapy exercises in subacromial impingement syndrome: a systematic review and meta-analysis". Seminars in Arthritis and Rheumatism, vol. 42, no. 3, pp. 297-316.

(172). Holmgren, T., Oberg, B., Sjoberg, I. & Johansson, K. 2012. "Supervised strengthening exercises versus home-based movement exercises after arthroscopic acromioplasty: a randomized clinical trial". Journal of Rehabilitation Medicine, vol. 44, no. 1, pp. 12-18.

(173).Desmeules, F., Cote, C.H. & Fremont, P. 2003. "Therapeutic exercise and orthopedic manual therapy for impingement syndrome: a systematic review". Clinical Journal of Sport Medicine:Official Journal of the Canadian Academy of Sport Medicine, vol. 13, no. 3, pp. 176-182.

(174). Kelly, S.M., Wrightson, P.A. & Meads, C.A. 2010. "Clinical outcomes of exercise in the management of subacromial impingement syndrome: a systematic review". Clinical Rehabilitation, vol. 24, no. 2, pp. 99-109.

(175). Santamato, A., Solfrizzi, V., Panza, F., Tondi, G., Frisardi, V., Leggin, B.G., Ranieri, M. & Fiore, P. 2009. "Short-term effects of high-intensity laser therapy versus ultrasound therapy in the treatment of people with subacromial impingement syndrome: a randomized clinical trial". Physical Therapy, vol. 89, no. 7, pp. 643-652.

(176).Dogan, S.K., Ay, S. & Evcik, D. 2010. "The effectiveness of low laser therapy in subacromial impingement syndrome: a randomized placebo controlled double-blind prospective study". Clinics, vol. 65, no. 10, pp. 1019-1022.

(177). Kurtais Gursel, Y., Ulus, Y., Bilgic, A., Dincer, G. & van der Heijden, G.J. 2004. "Adding ultrasound in the management of soft tissue disorders of the shoulder: a randomized placebo-controlled trial". Physical Therapy, vol. 84, no. 4, pp. 336-343.

(178). Calis, H.T., Berberoglu, N. & Calis, M. 2011. "Are ultrasound, laser and exercise superior to each other in the treatment of subacromial impingement syndrome? A randomized clinical trial". European Journal of Physical and Rehabilitation Medicine, vol. 47, no. 3, pp. 375-380.

(179).Aktas, I., Akgun, K. & Cakmak, B. 2007. "Therapeutic effect of pulsed electromagnetic field in conservative treatment of subacromial impingement syndrome". Clinical Rheumatology, vol. 26, no. 8, pp. 1234-1239.

(180).Bron, C., de Gast, A., Dommerholt, J., Stegenga, B., Wensing, M. & Oostendorp, R.A. 2011. "Treatment of myofascial trigger points in patients with chronic shoulder pain: a randomized, controlled trial". BMC Medicine, vol. 9, pp. 8.

(181).Green, S., Buchbinder, R. & Hetrick, S. 2005. "Acupuncture for shoulder pain". Cochrane Database of Systematic Reviews, vol. (2), no. 2, pp. CD005319.

(182). Guerra de Hoyos, J.A., Andres Martin Mdel, C., Bassas y Baena de Leon,E., Vigara Lopez, M., Molina Lopez, T., Verdugo Morilla, F.A. & Gonzalez Moreno, M.J. 2004. "Randomised trial of long term effect of acupuncture for shoulder pain". Pain, vol. 112, no. 3, pp. 289-298.

(183). Molsberger, A.F., Schneider, T., Gotthardt, H. & Drabik, A. 2010. "German Randomized Acupuncture Trial for chronic shoulder pain (GRASP) – a pragmatic, controlled, patientblinded, multi-centre trial in an outpatient care environment". Pain, vol. 151, no. 1, pp. 146- 154.

(184). Johansson, K., Bergstrom, A., Schroder, K. & Foldevi, M. 2011. "Subacromial corticosteroid injection or acupuncture with home exercises when treating patients with subacromial impingement in primary care – a randomized clinical trial". Family Practice, vol. 28, no. 4, pp. 355-365.

(185). Moraes, V.Y., Lenza, M., Tamaoki, M.J., Faloppa, F. & Belloti, J.C. 2014. "Platelet-rich therapies for musculoskeletal soft tissue injuries". The Cochrane Database of Systematic Reviews, vol. 4, pp. CD010071.

(186) Kesikburun, S., Tan, A.K., Yilmaz, B., Yasar, E. & Yazicioglu, K. 2013. "Platelet-rich plasma injections in the treatment of chronic rotator cuff tendinopathy: a randomized controlled trial with 1-year follow-up". The American Journal of Sports Medicine, vol. 41, no. 11, pp. 2609-2616.

(187). Rha, D.W., Park, G.Y., Kim, Y.K., Kim, M.T. & Lee, S.C. 2013. "Comparison of the therapeutic effects of ultrasound-guided platelet-rich plasma injection and dry needling in rotator cuff disease: a randomized controlled trial". Clinical Rehabilitation, vol. 27, no. 2, pp. 113-122.

(188). Husby, T., Haugstvedt, J.R., Brandt, M., Holm, I. & Steen, H. 2003. "Open versus arthroscopic subacromial decompression: a prospective, randomized study of 34 patients followed for 8 years". Acta Orthopaedica Scandinavica, vol. 74, no. 4, pp. 408-414.

(189).Donigan, J.A. & Wolf, B.R. 2011. "Arthroscopic subacromial decompression: acromioplasty versus bursectomy alone – does it really matter? A systematic review". The Iowa Orthopaedic Journal, vol. 31, pp. 121-126.
(190). Aydin, A., Yildiz, V., Kalali, F., Yildirim, O.S., Topal, M. & Dostbil, A. 2011, "The role of acromion morphology in chronic subacromial impingement syndrome", Acta Orthopaedica Belgica, vol. 77, no. 6, pp. 733-736.

(191).Budoff, J.E., Rodin, D., Ochiai, D. & Nirschl, R.P. 2005. "Arthroscopic rotator cuff debridement without decompression for the treatment of tendinosis". Arthroscopy: The Journal ofArthroscopic & Related Surgery, vol. 21, no. 9, pp. 1081-1089.

(192). Ellman, H. & Kay, S.P. 1991. "Arthroscopic subacromial decompression for chronic impingement. Two- to five-year results". The Journal of Bone and Joint Surgery. British volume, vol. 73, no. 3, pp. 395-398.
(193) Hermann Kay-Geert A, Backhaus Marina, Schneider Udo, Labs Karsten, Loreck Dieter, Zu¨ hlsdorf Svenda, et al. Rheumatoid arthritis of the shoulder joint: Comparison of conventional radiography, ultrasound, and dynamic contrast-enhanced magnetic resonance imaging. Arthritis Rheumatism 2003Dec;48(12):3338–49.

(194) McQueen FM. A vital clue to deciphering bone pathology: MRI bone edemas in rheumatoid arthritis and osteoarthritis. Ann Rheum Dis 2007;66(12):1549–52.
(195) McFarland EG, Selhi HS, Keyurapan E. Clinical evaluation of impingement: what to do and what works. J Bone Joint Surg Am 2006;88:432–41.

(196) John O'Neill MD. Musculoskeletal ultrasound; anatomy and Technique (ed); 2008. XII 348p.500illus.

(197) Khoury V, Cardinal E. Atrophy and fatty infileration of the supraspinatous muscle: Sonography versus MRI. AJR 2008;190:1105–11.

(198) Bureau NJ, Beauchamp M, Cardinal E, Brassard P. Dynamic sonography evaluation of the shoulder impingement syndrome. AJR 2006;187(1):216–20.

(199). Cone RO 3rd, Resnick D, Danzig L. Shoulder impingement syndrome: radiographic evaluation. Radiology 1984;150:29–33.

(200). Hardy DC, Vogler JB, White RH. The shoulder impingement syndrome: prevalence of radiographic findings and correlation with response to therapy. AJR Am J Roentgenol 1986;147:557-561.

(201). Bigliani LU, Ticker JB, Flatlow EL, et al. The relationship of acromial architecture to rotator cuff disease. Clin Sports Med 1991;10:823–838.

(202).. Peh WC, Farmer TH, Totty WG. Acromial arch shape: assessment with MR imaging. Radiology 1995;195:501–505.

(203). Bloom RA. The active abduction view: a new maneuver in the diagnosis of rotator cuff tears. Skeletal Radiol 1991;20:255–258.

(204). Kotzen LM. Roentgen diagnosis of rotator cuff tear: report of 48 surgically proven cases. Am J Roentgenol Radium Ther Nucl Med 1971;112: 507-511.

(205). De Smet AA, Ting YM. Diagnosis of rotator cuff tear on routine radiographs. J Can Assoc Radiol 1977;28:54-57.

(206). Pearsall AW 4th, Bonsell S, Heitman RJ, et al. Radiographic findings associated with symptomatic rotator cuff tears. J Shoulder Elbow Surg 2003;12: 122–127.

(207). Umans HR, Pavlov H, Berkowitz M, Warren RF. Correlation of radiographic and arthroscopic findings with rotator cuff tears and degenerative joint disease. J Shoulder Elbow Surg 2001;10:428-433.

(208) Jacobson JA. Shoulder US: anatomy, technique, and scanning pitfalls. Radiology2011;260(1):6-1.

.(209) Klauser AS, Tagliafico A, Allen GM, Boutry N, Campbell R, Court-Payen M, et al.Clinical indications for musculoskeletal ultrasound: a Delphi-based consen-sus paper of the European Society of Musculoskeletal Radiology. Eur Radiol2012;22(5):1140-8.

.(210) Martinoli C, Bianchi S, Prato N, Pugliese F, Zamorani MP, Valle M, et al.US of the shoulder: non-rotator cuff disorders. Radiographics 2003;23(2):381-401

.(211) Teefey SA, Hasan SA, Middleton WD, Patel M, Wright RW, Yamaguchi K.Ultrasonography of the rotator cuff: a comparison of ultrasonographic andarthroscopic findings in one hundred consecutive cases. J Bone Joint Surg Am2000;82(4):498–504.

.(212) Vlychou M, Dailiana Z, Fotiadou A, Papanagiotou M, Fezoulidis IV, MalizosK. Symptomatic partial rotator cuff tears: diagnostic performance of ultra-sound and magnetic resonance imaging with surgical correlation. Acta Radiol2009;50(1):101-5

(213) Singh JP. Shoulder ultrasound: what you need to know. Indian J Radiol Imaging2012;22(4):284–92.

(214) Nathalie J, Marc B, Etienne C. Dynamic sonography evaluation of shoulder impingement syndrome. AJR 2006;187:216–20.

(215) Hyun Ah Kim, Su, Ho Kim, Young-Il Seo. Ultrasonographic findings of the shoulder in patients with rheumatoid arthritis andcomparison with physical examination. J Korean Med Sci 2007;22(4):660-6.

(216). Naredo AE, Aguado P, Padr_on M, et al. A comparative study of ultrasonography with magnetic resonance imaging in patients with painful shoulder. J Clin Rheumatol 1999;5:184e92.

(217).. Huijsmans PE, Pritchard MP, Berghs BM, et al. Arthroscopic rotator cuff repair with double-row fixation. J Bone Joint Surg Am 2007;89: 1248e57.

(218) Read John W, Perko Mark. Ultrasound diagnosis of the subacromial impingement for lesions of the rotator cuff. AJUM 2010;13(2):11–5.

(219).Lee KS, Rosas HG. Musculoskeletal ultrasound: how to treat calcific tendinitis of the rotator cuff by ultrasound-guided single-needle lavage technique. AJR Am J Roentgenol 2010;195:638.

(220).. Serafini G, Sconfienza LM, Lacelli F, Silvestri E, Aliprandi A, Sardanelli F. Rotator cuff calcific tendonitis: short-term and 10-year outcomes after two-needle US-guided percutaneous treatment-nonrandomized controlled trial. Radiology 2009;252:157-64.

(221).Chaipat, L. & Palmer, W.E. 2006. "Shoulder magnetic resonance imaging". Clinics in Sports Medicine, vol. 25, no. 3, pp. 371-386.

(222).Cook, T.S., Stein, J.M., Simonson, S. & Kim, W. 2011. "Normal and variant anatomy of the shoulder on MRI". Magnetic Resonance Imaging Clinics of North America, vol. 19, no. 3, pp. 581-594.

(223).Sharma, P., Morrison, W.B. & Cohen, S. 2013. "Imaging of the shoulder with arthroscopic correlation". Clinics in Sports Medicine, vol. 32, no. 3, pp. 339-359.

(224).Rudez, J. & Zanetti, M. 2008. "Normal anatomy, variants and pitfalls on shoulder MRI". European Journal of Radiology, vol. 68, no. 1, pp. 25-35.

(225).Motamedi, D., Everist, B.M., Mahanty, S.R. & Steinbach, L.S. 2014. "Pitfalls in shoulder MRI: part 1 – normal anatomy and anatomic variants". AJR. American Journal of Roentgenology, vol. 203, no. 3, pp. 501-507.

(226).Vahlensieck, M. 2000. "MRI of the shoulder". European Radiology, vol. 10, no. 2, pp. 242-249.

(227).Fitzpatrick, D. & Walz, D.M. 2010. "Shoulder MR imaging normal variants and imaging artifacts". Magnetic Resonance Imaging Clinics of North America, vol. 18, no. 4, pp. 615-632.

(228).Ardic, F., Kahraman, Y., Kacar, M., Kahraman, M.C., Findikoglu, G. & Yorgancioglu, Z.R. 2006. "Shoulder impingement syndrome: relationships between clinical, functional, and radiologic findings". American Journal of Physical Medicine & Rehabilitation, vol. 85, no. 1, pp. 53-60.

(229).Theodoropoulos, J.S., Andreisek, G., Harvey, E.J. & Wolin, P. 2010. "Magnetic resonance imaging and magnetic resonance arthrography of the shoulder: dependence on the level of training of the performing radiologist for diagnostic accuracy". Skeletal Radiology, vol. 39, no. 7, pp. 661-667.

(230).La Rocca Vieira, R., Rybak, L.D. & Recht, M. 2012. "Technical update on magnetic resonance imaging of the shoulder". Magnetic Resonance Imaging Clinics of North America, vol. 20, no. 2, pp. 149-161, ix.

(231).Magee, T., Williams, D. & Mani, N. 2004. "Shoulder MR arthrography: which patient group benefits most?".AJR. American Journal of Roentgenology, vol. 183, no. 4, pp. 969-974.

(232).Schulte-Altedorneburg, G., Gebhard, M., Wohlgemuth, W.A., Fischer, W., Zentner, J., Wegener, R., Balzer, T. & Bohndorf, K. 2003. "MR arthrography: pharmacology, efficacy and safety in clinical trials". Skeletal Radiology, vol. 32, no. 1, pp. 1-12.

(233).Ozaki, J., Fujimoto, S., Nakagawa, Y., Masuhara, K. & Tamai, S. 1988. "Tears of the rotator cuff of the shoulder associated with pathological changes in the acromion. A study in cadavera". The Journal of Bone and Joint Surgery. American volume, vol. 70, no. 8, pp. 1224-1230.

(234).Nicholson, G.P., Goodman, D.A., Flatow, E.L. & Bigliani, L.U. 1996. "The acromion: morphologic condition and age-related changes. A study of 420 scapulas". Journal of Shoulder and ElbowSurgery, vol. 5, no. 1, pp. 1-11.

(235).Shah, N.N., Bayliss, N.C. & Malcolm, A. 2001. "Shape of the acromion: congenital or acquired – a macroscopic, radiographic, and microscopic study of acromion". Journal of Shoulder andElbow Surgery, vol. 10, no. 4, pp. 309-316.

(236).Saupe, N., Pfirrmann, C.W., Schmid, M.R., Jost, B., Werner, C.M. & Zanetti, M. 2006. "Association between rotator cuff abnormalities and reduced acromiohumeral distance". Americanjournal of roentgenology, vol. 187, no. 2, pp. 376-382.

(237).White, E.A., Schweitzer, M.E. & Haims, A.H. 2006. "Range of normal and abnormal subacromial/ subdeltoid bursa fluid". Journal of Computer Assisted Tomography, vol. 30, no. 2, pp. 316- 320.

.(238).Juul-Kristensen, B., Bojsen-Moller, F., Finsen, L., Eriksson, J., Johansson, G., Stahlberg, F. & Ekdahl, C. 2000a. "Muscle sizes and moment arms of rotator cuff muscles determined by magnetic resonance imaging". Cells, Tissues, Organs, vol. 167, no. 2-3, pp. 214-222.

(239).Juul-Kristensen, B., Bojsen-Moller, F., Holst, E. & Ekdahl, C. 2000b. "Comparison of muscle sizes and moment arms of two rotator cuff muscles measured by ultrasonography and magnetic resonance imaging". European Journal of Ultrasound, vol. 11, no. 3, pp. 161-173.

(240).Lehtinen, J.T., Tingart, M.J., Apreleva, M., Zurakowski, D., Palmer, W. & Warner, J.J. 2003. "Practical assessment of rotator cuff muscle volumes using shoulder MRI". Acta OrthopaedicaScandinavica, vol. 74, no. 6, pp. 722-729.

(241).Tingart, M.J., Apreleva, M., Lehtinen, J.T., Capell, B., Palmer, W.E. & Warner, J.J. 2003. "Magnetic resonance imaging in quantitative analysis of rotator cuff muscle volume". Clinical Orthopaedics and Related Research, vol. (415), no. 415, pp. 104-110.

(242).Holzbaur, K.R., Murray, W.M., Gold, G.E. & Delp, S.L. 2007. "Upper limb muscle volumes in adult subjects". Journal of Biomechanics, vol. 40, no. 4, pp. 742-749.

(243).Vidt, M.E., Daly, M., Miller, M.E., Davis, C.C., Marsh, A.P. & Saul, K.R. 2012. "Characterizing upper limb muscle volume and strength in older adults: a comparison with young adults". Journal of Biomechanics, vol. 45, no. 2, pp. 334-341.

(244).Tawfik, A.M., El-Morsy, A. & Badran, M.A. 2014. "Rotator cuff disorders: How to write a surgically relevant magnetic resonance imaging report?". World Journal of Radiology, vol. 6, no. 6, pp. 274-283.

(245).Goutallier, D., Postel, J.M., Bernageau, J., Lavau, L. & Voisin, M.C. 1994. "Fatty muscle degeneration in cuff ruptures. Pre- and postoperative evaluation by CT scan". Clinical Orthopaedics and Related Research, vol. (304), no. 304, pp. 78-83.